CH

D0461683

Westminster Public Library
3705 W 112th Ave
Westminster CO 80031
DISCARD
www.westminsterlibrary.org

she-ology

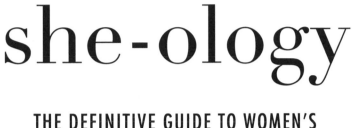

she-ology

THE DEFINITIVE GUIDE TO WOMEN'S INTIMATE HEALTH. PERIOD.

Sherry A. Ross, MD

Foreword by Reese Witherspoon

A SAVIO REPUBLIC BOOK

She-ology:
The Definitive Guide to Women's Intimate Health. Period.
© 2017 by Sherry A. Ross, MD
All Rights Reserved

ISBN: 978-1-68261-240-8
ISBN (eBook): 978-1-68261-241-5

No part of this book may be reproduced, stored in a retrieval system, or transmitted by any means without the written permission of the author and publisher.

The data for the chart on page 185 was compiled by ABC News.

Cover Design by Quincy Avilio
Illustrations by Megumi Wada
Interior Design and Composition by Greg Johnson/Textbook Perfect

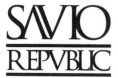

SAVIO
REPVBLIC

Published in the United States of America

TABLE OF CONTENTS

For my parents, Lorraine and Martin Ross, who have always encouraged me to dream big and reach for the stars, your love, inspiration and support knows no bounds.

In memory of my sister, Deena.

Throughout this book, you will see this symbol **VVL**, which represents my Visual Vaginal Library, or VVL. This is a library of images housed on my website that show women (and men) how different vaginal conditions look, up close and personal. For those readers who are interested, these images may be fascinating, scary, and captivating—all at the same time. They may help you to visualize these conditions if you choose to do a little more research. When you see the **VVL** you can visit **https://www.drsherry.com/visual-vaginal-library/** for images relating to the text.

INTRODUCTION

Vagina. Cooch. Va Jay Jay.

Don't look away. Even if you blush, that's okay. Seriously, I want to talk about this. I mean, what's a girl gotta do around here to get a little respect? We had our own one-woman play, *Vagina Monologues* by the brilliant Eve Ensler. We've been celebrated by artists and poets and pornographers for centuries, and yet, talking about the mighty V outside of doctor's offices and bedrooms has remained a major taboo. I think that's wrong. And I think it's time for a change, yesterday. Here's the thing. A healthy and confident vagina is a beautiful thing, the seat of our power, our sexuality, and our ability to create life. And a vagina that needs a little attention—medical, emotional, or good old-fashioned common sense—is nothing to inspire shame. It's part of the cycle of our lives, how we grow and mature into the many stages of our femininity. So why not embrace it, love it, wax it—or actively choose not to and let the big bush really come back into style—and above all else, *talk* about it, with our doctors, our partners, and among ourselves?

I've always been interested in hearing the stories of those who went unnoticed by most other people—even back in elementary school, I was drawn to the skinny, quiet boy with

glasses or the overweight girl who hid behind her bangs. I
courted these outsiders to be my friends because they seemed
so much more compelling than the flashier, more popular kids
in my class. From an equally young age, I knew I was going
to be a doctor (after I outgrew my original desire to be Barbra
Streisand). I went on rounds with my physician father as a
little girl, and not just for the free donuts. When I was pre-med
in college, I initially thought I would be a psychiatrist. But by
the time I did my residency at USC, I'd found my real calling:
Obstetrics and Gynecology, and more specifically, the path to
empowering my fellow women, one vagina at a time.

I guess you could say vagina power is my life's work. I've
been an OB-GYN for twenty-four years now, twenty-eight if
you count my four-year residency at USC. I consider it the
best job in the world because I get to talk to women every
day about all aspects of their health and wellbeing, vaginas
and all. I get to hear about the children I delivered now going
off to college. Not to mention all of the heartfelt accounts of
family reunions and fifty-year wedding anniversaries, and the
tragic stories of infidelities and sudden deaths, all of which
have become important to how I physically, and emotionally,
care for my patients. That's exactly why I love what I do: it
allows me to be there for women of all ages, medically and
non-medically. Also, I get to bring life into the world. There is
literally no greater moment than handing a baby to its mother,
father, or mother(s). After twenty-eight years of baby delivering, I still tear up.

So, yes, nothing is more important to me than women, and
my approach to their care is holistic to say the least. When
I see my patients, many of whom have been coming to me
for more than twenty-four years, my real concern is what

happened with their controlling mother-in-law, their daughter with the eating disorder, or their husband with the midlife crisis who wants a trial separation. Connecting with women and their families, and being their emotional support and sounding board, is not only my favorite part of my job. It's also how I help women to take care of themselves and stay healthy in all aspects of their lives. Thanks to my decades of experience, I know what questions to ask and what suggestions to make, in order to help women achieve their optimum physical and emotional health.

From my perspective, our vaginas are everything. I mean they are one of the most crucial parts of achieving real wellbeing, as they are a metaphor for who we are. And yet, as of right now, many of us can barely choke out the word. I've seen it again and again. Even in the privacy of my examining room, with the door closed, and no one there but my patient and me, so many women can't say vagina, or ask me their real questions about their body and how it interacts with their lives.

Whether these bashful vaginas result from outdated attitudes in our culture, or are partly responsible for creating societal norms, it's even worse outside my examining room. With porn on the rise, vaginas are everywhere. And yet, no one seems to want to admit how this new prevalence, and its resulting misconceptions about sex and the vagina is—or isn't—changing our romantic and sexual relationships and our relationships to our bodies and ourselves.

At the same time, our approach to vaginas in our society is undeniably juvenile. In June 2012, a bill was presented on the House floor seeking to regulate the use of the word "vagina" after Michigan Representative Lisa Brown was banned from speaking because she used the term in a debate over an anti-abortion bill.

"Brown's comment was so offensive, I don't even want to say it in front of women," complained Representative Mike Callton (R: Michigan). "I would not say that in mixed company."

Really? I'm astounded a ban would even be considered on a word that is, technically, a medical term. Also, in a larger sense, it defines women. I can't help but see this as a deliberate suppression of women, even just metaphorically, and feel inspired to fight back. In the course of writing this book, I realized how resistant mainstream media outlets are to having the word "vagina" said aloud on the airways. How can we best take care of our bodies and ourselves if we can't even say the word? Let's change that reality in the name of women's health, especially since there doesn't seem to be a problem in mainstream advertising for the treatment of erectile dysfunction!

All of this has led me to wonder why we're so squeamish about the term vagina, and what we can do to reclaim the word—and the vagina itself—while also taking back our bodies for our health, pleasure, and sense of personal power. I'm talking about an uprising here, ladies! Thankfully, there is some good news on this front. I spend the majority of my day with women, and I'm thrilled by a developing trend: many of my patients are now forward-thinking ladies who want to empower themselves and their vaginas. It's simply a matter of giving ourselves permission to go there, which more and more women are now willing to do.

I see a small version of this vagina revolution happening in my office every day—the truth is a lot of women enjoy coming to see me. I know. I know. You're saying: who actually likes going to the gynecologist? Well, wouldn't you, if it was a safe place for you to ask any question on your mind, talk openly about your relationship, or lack thereof, the stresses in your work and family life, and yes, of course, give your vagina the attention and care it deserves? Sadly, most women lack this in their lives—a little high-quality, adult "me" time. But I've watched it happen again and again: once we change our perspective and approach, it's possible to turn shame and anxiety into pride and a new sense of comfort and ease in our bodies.

I totally get why many of you consider it a toss-up between which is worse: going to the dentist, or coming to see me. Even though I don't run my office this way, I know very well what a trip to the OB-GYN is generally like. There's a rushed, in-and-out (literally!) sort of feeling, the sense of limited time and attention, of other patients waiting to be attended to behind other closed doors. The doctor hurries in, barely makes eye contact as he tries to absorb as much of your chart as possible, and drives the conversation in a narrow, mundane way: "How are your periods? Any problems? Okay, great, now scooch down."

And then the exam is happening, and sure, the oversized speculum may feel intrusive and uncomfortable, but soon enough it's over, and then you don't have to think about it for another year. Right there is a prime moment when an honest, open conversation could change everything: did you even know speculums come in different sizes, and you can ask for the small one to be used during your pelvic exam? Probably not. And why? Because you've always been too shy, or too ashamed, or even just too rushed, to have a real, meaningful talk with your doctor.

Which is why I make such a point to *really* talk with all of my female patients during our appointments, giving them the information they need to be both healthy and sexually satisfied. Often I invite their spouse or partner to join the conversation if I think it could be helpful. I'm more than happy to bridge the gaps for other doctors whenever I can. It happens so often. Every time I'm at a cocktail party, at least one—if not two—women pull me aside and ask me the questions they don't have time to ask their gyno. Or even if they *do* have the time in their appointment, these are the topics they can't bring themselves to discuss because they haven't had a good rapport with their doctor, or they're self-conscious about having a meaningful conversation during their exam

Usually, the cocktail party questioning begins with some variation of, "I hope this doesn't seem inappropriate or out of line." And then that first question will inevitably lead into a complete consultation.

"Why does sex hurt so much lately?"

"Why does my boyfriend say I have a funny new odor during oral sex?"

"Should I have my son get the HPV vaccine along with my daughter?"

Quite honestly, I don't mind these questions at all. In fact, I welcome them because women *need* this information. And unfortunately, with financial cutbacks and changes in our healthcare system, women have less and less time with their doctors during their routine exams. And with all of these constraints, sadly, the chance for any meaningful communication between doctors and their patients is being lost. My transferring patients have told me, time and again, about their awful experiences with past doctors who didn't listen or let them talk.

I feel strongly that we doctors have to lead the fight to bring back communication with our patients. This is why, in

Introduction

addition to authoring this book, I've founded Cycl (myCycl. com), a comprehensive and candid health and wellness platform for women by women. We need a dialogue, a community, a campaign, which is why I plan on creating a movement through this book, Cycl and my related blogs in order to make women feel heard and supported. Everything is connected: in life, in love, and in medicine. So let's take the conversation back for ourselves. Let's say the awkward words and ask the hard questions. It's okay to blush or giggle or be totally serious. We can also have a good time. Make it a party. All that matters is that we create a dialogue with each other about our vaginas and ourselves. That's exactly what I aim to do with my first book: provide all of the useful information I know women want and need, while sharing the relaxed, open and—yes, fun—environment I've created in my examining room.

I grew up with *Our Bodies, Ourselves* which was helpful but didn't dive into the most sensitive and surprisingly taboo issues of women's health. I want this book to be the new gold standard in women's wellness. I'm talking about a space where nothing, and I mean *nothing*, is off limits and everything is up for discussion. Let me tell you, as a woman who weathered an unsuccessful decade-long marriage to the father of my three sons, before finding true love with my wife of ten years, I've lived a lot in my lifetime. All of that is brought to bear in the compassion and advice I give my patients. There is no body-image issue, no medical condition, no emotional foible, and quite simply no vagina that is not welcome here.

Let's get into it. Let's get real. I've learned in twenty-four years of private practice: women have very different bodies, turn-ons and lives, but fundamentally, we all want the same things: to love and be loved, and to feel healthy and strong in our bodies, so we can share all we have to offer with those around us—our partners, our families, our coworkers, our communities. I wrote this book to let you know that you're all beautiful and of value in your own, unique ways. There is *absolutely* nothing to be ashamed of, ever, in any moment of your life, naked or fully clothed.

In coming up with the title of this book, I wanted a straightforward reference to what is, inarguably, the most famous of *female* genitalia. *She-ology* is a book for, in deference to, and in celebration of all people who have vaginas, no matter their gender identity, as well as all those without vaginas who desire more understanding of that most wondrous organ.

In drawing from my decades of experience as a doctor, I learned not only what this book should cover, I learned how best to address the most common questions from my practice. More often than not, these questions—and the patients I see—fall into obvious, distinct categories, which is why I've approached the V from the perspective of eighteen clear (and sometimes humorous) descriptives. Over the years, I've come to see vaginas as unique individuals that have different stages—sometimes simultaneously—just like the women to whom they belong. While there is some overlap, most women are specifically focused on their vagina's current moment and may not have much need to look backwards or forwards. Others are curious about what's ahead, or may be looking back to begin educating a daughter, niece or goddaughter about what to expect as she herself becomes a woman. Anyone with a vagina and anyone who loves someone with a vagina needs to read this book.

With all of this in mind, the book is divided by vagina type, with eighteen sections in all, from the adolescent

Introduction

("Tween") vagina, to the divorced vagina, all the way through the menopausal vagina (otherwise known as "The Mature V"), with some detours in between to address the kinds of issues women *really* want to know about—including Adventurous, Bashful, Sporty, and Perfect vaginas.

This way, it's possible to flip directly to the section that will address your specific issue or question. Once there, you can learn about the experiences my patients have had in this area over the years, so you'll know you're not alone, and you'll see how my patients and I have successfully dealt with this very subject in the past. You'll find all of the highly specific, completely accurate medical advice you won't find from a blind Internet search, written in the conversational tone of someone who cares about you and your vagina. This is me, not only a doctor, but also your soul sister, and as I've already made clear, we're in this together, and we're going to make this enjoyable.

I guess you could say I've got a vagina agenda, and we're not going to stop until we've launched a full-on revolt. Which is the other way to read this book—as a form of uprising in and of itself. Sit down and enjoy it from start to finish, learn about your vagina, learn about your sisters' vaginas, and by doing so, learn about yourself. It will be time well spent, believe me. Not only will you feel more at home in your body, you'll feel more empowered and alive. That, right there, is the magical power of the vagina, and it's only getting stronger, but only if we choose to make it so. Let's do it. Let the dialogue begin. *Viva la revolution. Viva la vagina.* The Vagina Revolution is ON!

A NOTE ABOUT THE BOOK'S TITLE, SHE-OLOGY

Although this book is about a Vagina Revolution, another revolution has been picking up much-needed steam for many years. As a woman who also happens to be a gynecologist, a lesbian, and an advocate for LGBTQ equality, I'm pleased to report that the Gender Revolution is also in progress right now. Simply put, the Gender Revolution seeks the acknowledgement and acceptance that gender is not a given, rather it is a choice, regardless of what is between one's legs.

In 2015 the American Dialect Society voted "they" as word of the year. "They," formerly used to mean more than one person, male or female, is now a widely accepted gender-neutral term for one or more persons. The gender binary system, a categorization dependent upon the sex assigned to a person at birth, is slowly being replaced by gender identity, which is dictated by one's internal sense of identity—be it male, female, or something in between. In the wake of this acceptance of gender identity, incoming students at Harvard, Brown, Wesleyan and other influential universities are now asked to identify with a gender pronoun in which the choices have been expanded from She and He to They, Ze, E, Ev, Hir, Xe, Hen, Ve, Ne, Per, Thon, and Mx, and Facebook now offers more than fifty gender identity options for new users. Clearly, the general population is slowly catching on.

It is my hope that regardless of the pronoun you use to describe yourself, you may discover things in this book that will help you live a fuller, healthier and more informed life.

FOREWORD

Reese Witherspoon

When I was nine years old I figured out what my mother did for a living. I knew she was a nurse, but she'd started working at a new job with a new doctor. She would come home at night alternately exhausted and overjoyed.

One day I asked her, "Mommy, what do you do at work all day?"

She said, "I help ladies have babies."

I said, "Why do you have to help them have a baby?"

She said, "Because sometimes they can't have babies by themselves, and I am there to help them."

That's when I understood that my mother's life mission was to help other women.

My mom started working for one of the only fertility clinics in Nashville, Tennessee in the mid-1980s. When I was a little older, she told me about the woman who rejoiced when she finally got a positive result on a pregnancy test. She told me about the woman she held and cried with when a long-awaited pregnancy test turned out negative. She was on those women's journeys right with them. I listened to all my mother's stories with awe, intrigued by what she did to help women, not only medically, but also emotionally.

My mother worked in women's health care for more than thirty-five years. (To be honest, it was forty years, but she says that makes her sound too old.) I learned a lot from my mother about the importance of knowing about your body and of being unafraid to ask questions, and about being responsible for your own health care.

That's why, when it came to a time to find an OB-GYN to deliver my third child, I asked women I respected who they would recommend. One of my closest friends recommended Dr. Sherry Ross.

Now, one of the first things people should know about Dr. Sherry is that upon entering her office you're greeted with an entire wall covered in photos of women giving birth—babies in various states of afterbirth, little faces screaming as they come into the world and joyful pictures of Dr. Sherry holding newborns next to sweaty, enthusiastic new parents.

It's very brave to greet expectant couples with such realistic images, but those images are the truth of an OB-GYN's job.

Dr. Sherry is a lot like that wall. She is honest. She is thoughtful. She is brave. And she is on the front line of the revolution for women to talk about their health and welfare, starting at a young age.

Dr. Sherry and her nurse Dani held my hand through every stage of my third pregnancy—the hormonal tears, the joy of finding out I was having a healthy little boy, the exhaustion brought on by an extra 45 post-pregnancy pounds. They hugged me (and my husband) at every visit and they let me know everything was gonna be all right, that, actually, everything would be great!

Foreword

Honestly, I have never met a person more passionate about women's healthcare. I don't know where Dr. Sherry finds the time to personally text and send copious amounts of emails to all her patients about their specific health concerns. But she does.

Whether she is calming a nervous mother about a blood test or speaking with a teenager about birth control, Sherry's incredible bedside manner and her passion to help people understand their bodies is always evident.

So, naturally, I was thrilled when she called and told me she was writing a book about women's health. No one is more knowledgeable, in my opinion. No one cares more about women's health than Dr. Sherry Ross.

Except, maybe, my mother. But she is retired.

And by the way, *she* thinks the world of Dr. Sherry as well.

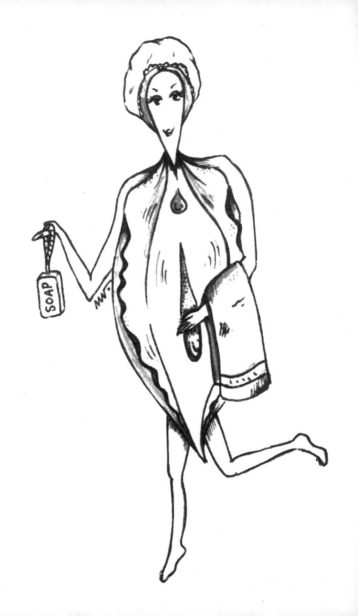

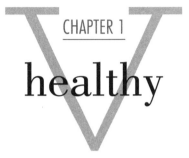

healthy

66 I was raised to always try to be the best version of myself mentally, emotionally, and physically. Performing was in my blood from an early age, so I was fortunate enough to have a mother who nurtured my love of singing and dancing. In fact, my sister and I grew up dancing, which made us naturally aware of every aspect of our bodies. The dancing world definitely had a big influence on us, and despite the tendencies for dancers to sometimes push too hard and neglect their health, our mother always encouraged us to take care of our bodies.

When I went through puberty, my body and metabolism changed in ways I wasn't prepared for. I was honestly confused as to why I suddenly couldn't eat ten of my mom's crispy mini pancakes on a Sunday anymore without gaining weight. If that wasn't bad enough, the surge of hormones affected my emotional and psychological state. My body was changing in ways that I felt I had no control over. It was definitely an eye-opening time for me, especially after being such a disciplined performer for so many years. Thankfully, my mother was able to help me through those difficult teen years, and I moved forward into some awesome experiences, not the least of which was appearing on *American Idol*.

Even though I didn't officially win *American Idol*, I felt like a winner as I realized that I'd become a role model for young women—a role that I take very seriously, especially in a world that is still predominantly run by men. I realized that it's up to my generation to change the outdated rules of society today.

Now, more than ever, I take care of my body. I eat a healthy, well-balanced diet, sleep at least seven hours a night, drink tons of water, and exercise regularly. I know "perfection" should never be one's goal because, basically, it doesn't exist!

I try not to overindulge in any one thing, except maybe classical music and the San Francisco 49ers. Since health is a priority, I see my gynecologist, Dr. Sherry, on a regular basis—she reminds me that "strong and healthy" trumps all.

I can't say I've tried some of the trends in vaginal cleaning, but I am a firm believer in daily hygiene—a non-fragrant soap and water has always worked well for me in the "housekeeping" department.

Because I've been fortunate enough to pursue my dreams, I want to encourage other young women to do the same. If I can serve as a role model for women to be true to who they are, to be healthy in body and mind—which definitely includes a healthy V—then I will really feel like I have accomplished something great. 99

—**Katharine McPhee** Actress, Singer, Songwriter

Healthy V

*My mother told me never to use soap on the vagina because
I could get a yeast infection. She said to just douche once a
month and that will take care of the cleaning. Is that true?
–Cheryl, age 32*

We women usually know what's best for our particular hair,
our teeth, our feet. Isn't *that* true? And if we don't know, we
experiment, we research, we **ask**. Likewise, we know the exact
contours of our necks, our chins, our fingernails. We notice
every new freckle, tic, and skin fold, but most women not only
have no idea what their vaginas look like, they don't know
what special care it takes to maintain them!

I still have patients, like Cheryl, parrot what their mothers
or grandmothers told them about taking care of that lone
vista *down south*. Old habits, especially the ones handed
down to us by our mothers, die hard. In my practice, I seldom
have anyone ask me about the best cleaning techniques for a
healthy vagina!

Healthy body, healthy mind, healthy soul...a healthy V is
metaphor for all three. As soon as I ask a patient to scootch
down on the exam table I know who is properly cleaning their
vagina—a non-fragrant soap and water, please—and who isn't.
In fact, I can tell a lot about a woman who cleans her vagina.
The ones who don't are usually detached emotionally and physically (to some extent) from their vajayjays. I'm the gyno; I can
tell all this during a pelvic exam. My eyes and nose don't lie.

Is the vagina really self-cleaning? –Claudia, age 29

Unfortunately, I always think of an oven when I hear the term
"self-cleaning," and the truth is, while heat is an oven-cleaning
friend, it is not for the vagina. In fact, heat and moisture buildup
on the vulva is a path to vaginal itching and irritation—which

is why it's important to change sanitary pads frequently and a good idea to choose cotton or cotton-crotch panties. Synthetic fibers (in both pads and panties) tend to trap heat and increase friction. But I digress, just a little...

As far as the miraculous "self-cleaning" ability of the vagina, it is partially true, but the regular use of a *non-fragrant soap and water* is not only safe, it is recommended. Vagisil and Summer's Eve both have intimate wash products especially formulated for the vagina that are the perfect choices for the daily cleaning a healthy V!

A healthy vagina needs the same attention to hygiene as any other part of your body. Between the urine and sweat and the close proximity to the anus, your vagina must be cleaned regularly in order to prevent dirt and bacterial buildup, and to avoid the unpleasant odors that may develop throughout the day. Debris builds up in the labia grooves from improper hygiene. This debris is commonly referred to as "smegma," a potent brew of shed skin cells, skin oils, and moisture, which can occur both in male and female genitalia. **VVL**

One of the most common organisms associated with bladder infections is E. Coli, which is no wonder given that the vagina and anus are in such close proximity. A good, easy practice to observe is to always wipe front to back after a bowel movement in order to avoid introducing any unwanted bowl flora, such as the pernicious E. Coli and Enterococcus bacteria. Genital wipes are also a good way of keeping the vagina and anus clean after bowel movements and urination.

During menstruation it's very important to change your tampons or sanitary pads at least every two to six hours, depending on the flow—generally more often on those heavy first and second days. A low absorbency tampon will minimize your risk for Toxic Shock Syndrome, a potentially fatal illness caused by a bacterial toxin. And no one should be using tampons on a regular basis to absorb discharge!

So, as a gynecologist, in direct opposition to mom's well-intentioned advice, I suggest that your **daily routine** involve *cleaning your vagina and labia as if it were any other part of your body.* Nothing more is needed than your hand and a *gentle, non-fragrant soap* (Dove, Caress, Aveeno, Cedaphil, and Eucerin are a few brands that come to mind) *or an intimate wash.* Scented soaps, cleaners and feminine grooming products can actually upset the normal pH balance of the vagina, causing infections and skin irritation. With that said, **douches** need not apply (literally...and figuratively).

Douching, which involves squirting a premade cleaning mixture high into the vagina, is basically useless. This type of internal vaginal cleaning does not—I repeat: *does not*—help to keep the vagina smelling fresh and clean. The active cleaning ingredients used in most douches can actually upset the healthy vaginal discharge and pH balance, thereby *creating* a yeast or bacterial infection.

A "Steaming" Trend

Long before Gwyneth Paltrow and other holistic health practitioners (often rooted in Southern California) started **vaginal steaming**, the Mayan women were undergoing the same treatment, as prescribed by their own traditional healers. The process involves sitting or squatting over a concentrated steam of mugwort and wormwood, which is believed to cleanse the uterus as well as the vagina. Practitioners believe that this helps in treating everything from irregular periods, to vaginal cysts, bladder infections, yeast infections, uterine fibroids, hemorrhoids, and even infertility.

My concern is that the consequences of steam cleaning are similar to those of douching. Too much internal cleaning is not a good thing. The vagina has its own internal wash cycle that keeps it clean and balanced. Steam and extreme heat, as well as douches and antibiotics, can disrupt the natural pH balance of the vagina, resulting in a yeast or bacterial infection.

An herbal steam on the outside of the vagina may have a relaxing and calming effect beneficial to vagina and mind, but the medical-research jury is still out as to any proven benefits of vaginal steaming.

Meanwhile, I plan on waiting to recommend this ancient steam clean to my patients.

Smells, Cells and Discharge, Courtesy of the Vagina

What's normal?

The vagina is equipped with more than thirty organisms that keep it acidic and free of infections. These organisms produce secretions (**discharge**) to naturally cleanse the vagina, much like the mouth does with saliva and the eyes do with tears. Normal discharge is simply a fluid that carries away dead cells and bacteria, protecting the vagina from infection. This healthy discharge will appear clear to milky in color and will have a "vagina-like" smell. The vagina is *not* meant to smell like a rose garden, but it does have its own familiar scent. Depending on the time of month, vaginal discharge can change in consistency and smell.

In between periods, typically around Day Fourteen, you may notice a clear, slippery, odorless discharge the consistency of egg whites. This is also completely normal, and it suggests *ovulation*. During *puberty* a milky discharge (leucorrhea) is produced. This naturally occurring discharge protects the stability of the vagina.

But what about all those other strange odors?

All of us vagina owners know how disconcerting it can be to encounter a new smell down south, so the key is to know what your particular "normal" smells like. Since the vagina is very sensitive to changes in your daily environment, anything that affects its pH balance will also affect the smell and consistency of discharge. Factors that affect this balance include:

* Antibiotic use
* Douching
* Spermicides
* New sexual partners
* Frequency of sexual intercourse
* Sex toys
* Hormonal imbalances such as pregnancy, breastfeeding, and menopause
* Jacuzzi jets aimed anywhere near the vagina
* Diet, stress, exercise, and weather changes

These factors may not only cause a strange new odor; they also may create other **uncomfortable symptoms** such as:

* Vulvar itching, burning, redness, and swelling
* Yellow or gray discharge that may vary in thickness and consistency

A strong, foul, fishy vaginal odor with a thin, grayish-white discharge is a classic symptom of bacterial infections, but it can also be a result of other types of **organisms** (infections) such as **Candidiasis, Bacterial Vaginosis/Gardnerella, Trichomoniasis, Chlamydia** and **Gonorrhea** (which I covered in greater detail in Benched V, Chapter 4).

If you experience any of the aforementioned symptoms, it is important that you see your healthcare provider. She can take a series of vaginal cultures in order to determine what organism is involved. Many women will invariably self-diagnose vaginal discharge and itching as a common yeast infection. I know it seems much easier to head to the drug store for an over-the-counter medication, but, unfortunately, you may only make your symptoms worse and delay a proper diagnosis and treatment. Vaginal cultures can confirm what organism is causing your disruptive symptoms in order for the best treatment to be prescribed. Even if you tend towards more "natural" remedies, please, before you start *packing yogurt* into your vagina, take a trip to your healthcare provider to check things out properly.

And as long as we're talking about "packing," I'd like to share a brief cautionary tale...

Adventures in Non-Organic Materials and the Vagina

Catherine is a precocious fifteen-year-old patient of mine. In her skin-tight True Religion jeans and three-inch heels, she also appears much older than fifteen, which is not surprising given that she floats in behind her equally precocious eighteen-year-old sister Melissa, who is also a patient of mine. The girls seat themselves across from me in my office, but before

Healthy V

I can utter a word I'm struck by an indescribably foul smell. Melissa blurts out, with her usual candor, "Catherine's pussy stinks! Something is definitely not right!" Catherine said she was clueless as to the cause. She showered regularly, was still a virgin, used tampons without difficulty, and she didn't have any other symptoms. I took Catherine into the exam room, without Big Sis, so that we could talk privately, and then I asked her if there was anything else I should know. There followed a silence you could drive a truck through before she answered, "A few months ago I took Melissa's favorite porn DVDs—*Grand Theft Orgy* and *Whorecraft*—and I watched women putting foreign objects into their vaginas, and it kind of looked interesting and exciting. Since I'm a virgin I thought I'd try it." Apparently Catherine had some small bouncing balls and had inserted four of them into her vagina. Aside from not having any "fun" with the activity, she was only able to remove three of the four. The last ball wasn't reachable, but she thought that it would just fall out...eventually. In the past four months, "eventually" had come and gone. Catherine was too embarrassed to tell anyone, especially her sister, despite the thick green discharge she was experiencing and the fact that the odor had grown so intense that her family had taken note of it. Of course, I followed right up with a pelvic exam, and low and behold, I could see the remnants of a partially disintegrated blue bouncy ball. After cleaning her vagina with Betadine and giving her antibiotics, I washed out the remaining pieces and placed them in a HAZMAT bag. My nurse, Dani, made a mad dash to dispose of the bag away from unsuspecting patients and staff. Luckily, there is a special place for things that are unimaginably malodorous.

News flash: The vagina is not a storage unit. *Obviously,* you say, but the truth is that we healthcare providers hear about women putting all sorts of unusual things in their vaginas—from guns to baggies of drugs, prescription pills, knives, and bouncy balls. In fact, recently a young woman named Shekira Thompson was arrested at JFK Airport for trying to transport $10,000 worth of cocaine in her vagina—apparently the half-pound of powder was concealed in an egg-shaped container inside her *Smuggler V.*

Note: as elastic and as good a hiding place as it may seem, the vagina simply doesn't do well with foreign objects, especially over long periods of time.

You and Your Gyno...a Lifetime Relationship

Regular visits to your gynecologist or healthcare provider should be part of your routine in maintaining a healthy vagina. A good time to begin this routine (and relationship) is between the ages of 13 and 15. At that juncture, a first visit should include discussions about menses, the HPV vaccine and any and all questions related to body, sex and overall gynecologic health—although, at that early age a visit would probably not include an internal pelvic exam unless there was a specific concern.

As per the current guidelines for **Pap testing**, women should have their first Pap test (or Pap smear) at age 21. Between the ages of 21 and 28 it's recommended that women be tested every three years. Women 30 to 65 should have a Pap and HPV (human papilloma virus) test every five years (or you can stick to your Pap test alone every three). Screening after 65 seems unnecessary if adequate prior screening has been negative and you're not deemed "high risk." **VVL**

Healthy V

Any screening of the cervix may also include a check for HPV, since this virus is directly associated with an increase in cervical cancer. The HPV vaccine has been proven to decrease the incidence of contracting HPV and is recommended for girls and boys around 11 or 12 years of age, although the targeted age group is nine to twenty-six, prior to the beginning of sexual activity. Even if you've already contracted HPV, you may still benefit from this vaccine.

Your gynecologist visit may also include screening for other sexually transmitted infections (STIs) including Chlamydia, Gonorrhea, Syphilis, genital warts (a possible symptom of HPV), Herpes Simplex Virus, HIV, and Hepatitis B. Ideally, you should be screened for STIs in between new partners.

You care for your hair and car (and kids) on a regular basis, so the same attention is necessary for that physical seat of your female being! I hope you're saying to yourself, "Well, since you put it *that* way!"

I do put it that way, in fact, while sipping a lemon-drop martini with my best girlfriend, after a long day in the exam room, I've blurted out, "please tell me you wash your vagina with a non-fragrant soap daily?" To which she's responded with a toast and a cry of "hell, yes!"

You probably wash your face daily. Do the same for your vagina, especially if you have a date with your gynecologist for your annual pelvic exam. Besides, you owe it to yourself to keep your vagina as healthy and cared for as possible. Maybe your mother was right when she told you to keep up appearances...that is, if she was referring to down south.

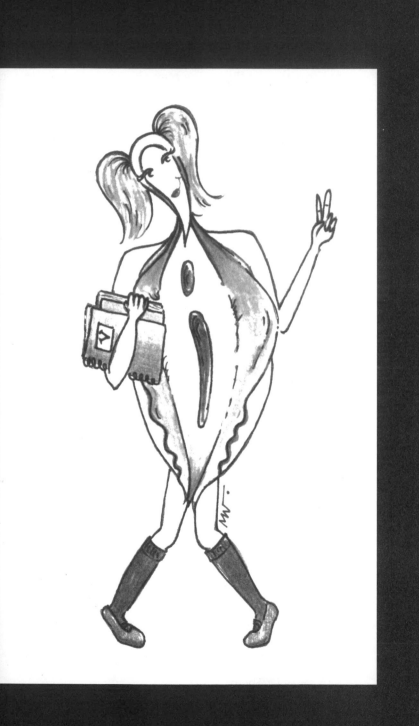

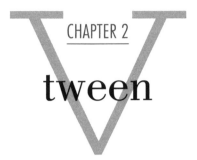

CHAPTER 2

tween

"Mother–daughter relationships can be challenging at times, but I have found fewer struggles with my girls by treating them with respect, valuing their opinions, and talking to them openly. I have always asked them to share in honesty so that I can support them best in their journey. We have learned to communicate with each other from a place of love, support, and compassion.

My personal health has taken me off course a number of times after being diagnosed with Lyme disease in 2012. It's been the most challenging and disruptive part of my life during these past few years. I have always prided myself on a healthy and holistic lifestyle, eating a clean diet, exercising regularly.

I have educated and inspired my girls to take care of themselves, physically, mentally and spiritually. I have always integrated Eastern medicine philosophies in my health care and so have my girls. I took them both to see Dr. Sherry to start forming their own relationship in their mid-teens. Even though we talked about what it meant to be sexually active, having safe sex, and being in touch with your body, I knew it was important for them to have an independent relationship with their doctor. I am not sure who was more nervous about their first gyno visit with Dr. Sherry, them or me. I was proud of them and knew this was the right step for them to feel safe and in control of their own personal health and wellness. Now they are comfortable enough to call or text Dr. Sherry directly knowing she will be there for them in my absence. They know I encourage healthy living and I want them to embrace this philosophy as well. 〞

—**Yolanda Hadid** Mother, TV Personality, Health Advocate
    Dedicated to Lyme Disease Awareness

Letitia has been my patient for two years. Once again, on referencing her chart, I've done a double-take as I realize that the poised, mature young woman before me is just seventeen. On her last visit she had to wait more than forty-five minutes for me as I'd been delayed by a delivery. It was okay, she told me, because she'd had time to jot down a bunch of questions that she'd been meaning to ask. Letitia was particularly inquisitive about her changing body, and she always gave me a run for my money in the questions department.

First she asked about the baby I'd delivered: What was his name? "Henry," I told her. Then she asked if I was ever freaked out during a delivery. I said, "I love what I do, so I rarely, if ever, get freaked out by delivering a baby. There's no moment as magical as delivering a baby and then handing that child over to its parents. There's nothing like it." Her eyes went wide in reaction. I waited. "Okay," she said.

Tween V

Then she launched into her laundry list of questions, the first of which was about a vaginal discharge and odor that she'd been noticing over the past couple months. Letitia was still a virgin, and she had never been sexual with a partner. She'd read enough to realize that she probably didn't have an infection because the discharge was colorless and she didn't have any itching or burning. "Should I be douching?" she asked, and then addressed all her concerns without a breath. "I'm really just curious about what's going on down there. What's the discharge? I read something about the vagina being 'self-cleaning.' I mean I'm cleaning myself with soap. Is that enough? I'm a little confused. And my friends keep talking about the Diva cup. What do you think about using that instead of tampons? A friend of mine couldn't get her tampon out!"

Adolescence. Remember it? You may have blocked it out, but what you can recall is a vague feeling of how difficult a time it was and how many new issues there were to contend with—environmental, social, financial, psychosocial. Ah, you remember now; at least it was never dull. Probably you had a lot of unanswered questions as well. Probably some of those questions had to do with your own body and sexuality, which is why you want to give your daughter the knowledge and encouragement to take control of her vagina (and her life) in order to empower herself on her own journey. Well, you've come to the right place, because I believe that our daughters are the front line of the vagina revolution.

She-ology

66 "E very year in America about 5 million girls get their first period, and about 10 million parents either talk to them about it or don't. That's the data. But I don't care much for data when it comes to menarche or puberty for that matter. What I care about are feelings.

As founder of HelloFlo I am in the unique position to hear from countless girls and their parents about what puberty and coming of age is like in the current landscape. And it's quite different than it was for me, a Gen-Xer. Today's girls generally know more about EVERYTHING. If they have a question, all they need to do is google it and they have a plethora of answers (and pictures).

This is why I've dedicated my past few years to putting honest, accurate, and relatable information online. Young women need to know about their bodies, and they need to learn the facts from trusted sources. And they have questions...lots of them. And it's our job to give them answers. That's why books like Dr. Sherry's are so critical. We need to know the answers so we can educate future generations of girls.

So read about the Tween V, talk to the girls you know, and make sure they know the magic of their bodies. Think of how lucky and healthy we'd all be if we all learned about our bodies and viewed them through the magical and positive lens of *She-ology*. 99

—**Naama Bloom** Founder of HelloFlo.com, Author

"Question Everything." –George Carlin

When it comes to talking to our teens about their sexual, reproductive and health behaviors it can be awkward for all parties involved—which is why I especially love when a teen like Stephanie gets to the point. Mostly, though, it's not easy for parents or their teens. Many parents, when they were teens themselves, didn't have the experience of healthy and open dialogues about these issues with their own parents, so they don't have a model for this type of dialogue. Where to start? Parents, healthcare providers, and even mentors need first to create a supportive environment for their teens to talk about sex and health issues, otherwise the important questions (and even the seemingly mundane ones) won't get asked.

A recent study out of Duke University Medical Center reported in *JAMA Pediatrics* showed that one third of teens did not ask questions about sex or discuss their sexual activity, sexuality, dating, or sexual identity during their yearly checkups. The same study showed that the topic of sex was brought up at 65 percent of all visits, but the conversations lasted an average of only *36 seconds!*

You may think the patients of mine who are mothers of teenagers would have no problem in transitioning their daughters from pediatric exams to gynecological ones, but many of the mothers I see worry that if they bring their daughters for an appointment and a realistic conversation about birth control, that alone is permission to become sexually active. Seeing a gynecologist is *not* a catalyst for teens to have sex; rather, it's an important step in screening, preventive services, and other healthcare guidance.

There's no avoiding the fact that every year some 750,000 adolescents between fifteen and nineteen become pregnant. Surprisingly, the teen pregnancy rate in the United States is one of the highest among industrialized nations—although the pregnancy rate for the fifteen to nineteen-year-old age group fell thirty-eight percent between 1990 and 2004, reaching its lowest rate since 1976. We may want to thank MTV's *16 and*

Pregnant and its *Teen Mom* sequel for the decline in the teen pregnancy rate. According to a National Bureau of Economic Research study, those shows alone have been thought to help lower teen birth rate by six percent, and may have prevented more than 20,000 births to young moms in 2010 alone. Chelsea Houska, 22, from *Teen Mom 2* confessed, "Having a baby made everything more difficult.... If we're scaring teens, that's good!". Special thanks to the Reality TV teen moms for serving as a reminder to us all.

However, pregnancy isn't the only concern amongst this age group.

Recently it has been shown that twenty-five percent of sexually active teens and young adults 15–24 acquire almost fifty percent of all new *sexually transmitted infections* (STIs). Because of screening programs that tend to focus more on females, the rate of STIs looks to be higher in women than men. Adolescents that use alcohol or drugs are more likely to have unplanned and unprotected sex, which put them at a higher risk for contracting STIs, and half of them surveyed said the main reason their peers don't use contraception is because of alcohol and drug use. Women ages fourteen to nineteen were also found to have a twenty-four percent prevalence of **HPV** (more on this preventable virus in **Healthy V**). The good news is the new Gardasil 9 HPV vaccine can prevent 90% of the HPV high-risk types causing cervical cancer including the scary four: Types 6, 11, 16 and 18. This is why I strongly suggest getting the vaccine at twelve or thirteen, *before* a young woman becomes sexually active.

Starting between the ages of 13 and 15, it's recommended girls visit a gynecologist for an initial consultation and a simple external examination. This "external-only" pelvic exam allows the doctor to evaluate the external genital anatomy, issues of personal hygiene, and look for any possible abnormalities of the vagina and vulva. This consultation should open the door to enlightening conversations about healthy behavior and health risks.

The earlier the dialogue begins, the better chance our teens have to avoid STIs, unwanted pregnancies, and alcohol, tobacco and drug use. In fact, the sooner the dialogue, the better the chance of a healthy *lifestyle*.

(As far as the question of "what's going on down there?" is concerned, a peek into the **Healthy V** chapter is a great place to start, since that's where we delve into the *care and maintenance of the healthy vagina*.)

An Alternative to Tampons

Diva cup certainly sounds a whole lot cooler than **menstrual cup**, but truth be told, it's simply a *brand* of menstrual cup—a handy feminine hygiene product designed to collect menstrual blood inside the vagina. Although inserting and extracting a menstrual cup is a bit more intimate an experience than most women want to have with their periods, the cup has grown in popularity. Some brands come in two sizes, small and large—the small for women who have not given birth, the large for, well, vaginas that have had babies pushed through them. If you've not had a baby, you would most certainly purchase a small size so as to avoid having the cup fall out when straining during intense exercise or when pooping.

Many different brands of menstrual cup are now available, all with similar qualities, including a construction of vag-safe material, such as plastic, silicone-based plastic, and latex (which is hypo-allergenic and biocompatible) that meets medical safety standards. Some cups are disposable, while other need only be replaced every couple of years.

If you're wondering whether the menstrual cup is for you, here are **The Top Six Things Women Love about the Menstrual Cup**:

* It's a natural and environmentally friendly way to collect Aunt Flo's monthly gift and a healthier alternative to commercially produced tampons.
* Tampons and Kotex pads are costly! You may only have to buy one menstrual cup a year, at an average cost of $40.
* Convenience. No need to stockpile tampons and pads (especially in that tiny, trendy purse you love).
* Menstrual cups are more comfortable than tampons and pads.
* Nighttime blood collection is often easier.
* You may use the cup to collect blood if you want to have sex during your period.

On the *con* side: It's not so easy to insert that cute little cup into the very back of the vagina. You may end up wondering: *Where is that third hand when I need it?* Same deal when removing the cup, which sometimes proves to be a challenging and bloody mess. Also, straining to poop can pop a cup from your vagina (need I say more?).

If the "pros" of the menstrual cup have sparked your interest, give it a try. Shop around and experiment with different brands in order to find the right fit for your vagina. With menstrual cups, as with sneakers and bras, one size does not fit all.

When a Tampon Signals Trouble

Sabrina was a fifteen-year-old virgin when she came to see me at a last minute appointment. In tenth grade at Costa Mesa High School, she was a model United Nations student and already a star soccer player on the varsity team. Sabrina nervously twisted her hair as she sat across from me. She was there because she was worried about what was happening in her vagina. "I tried a tampon for the first time, you know? And now I can't pull it out! It's a disaster! It was supposed to be so easy. So, I put in a small-sized one last night and now I can't get it out of my vagina!" It all made sense during the exam as I looked at Sabrina's outer vagina and noticed an extra piece of skin coming down from the twelve to six o'clock position. The diagnosis was a septate hymen, which meant that the tampon could not easily be removed because the opening to the vagina was separated by a septum (or band of tissue). I was able to remove the tampon, and then I scheduled Sabrina for a simple outpatient procedure to correct the problem. **VVL**

Not that I want to harp on the notion of a gynecological visit, (I will if I have to) but sometimes external vaginal exams can detect certain abnormalities.

A **septate hymen**, as the one experienced by Sabrina, is often the cause when a young girl has trouble inserting or removing a tampon. It may also be the cause of an irregular menstrual blood flow or pain with sex. In the case of a septate hymen an extra piece of tissue is seen at the entrance of the vagina, requiring surgical removal to correct the problem. This is also the case in a **partial imperforate hymen**, when the hymen is *partially blocked*. **VVL**

An **imperforate hymen** is a complete blockage of the entrance into the vagina. The diagnosis of an imperforate or partially imperforate hymen is usually made in puberty and occurs in one in a thousand girls. Period bleeding will back up in a complete blockage of the exit of the vagina. Pelvic pain may be the first sign of these abnormalities, usually around the age of eleven or twelve, when menses first begins. Treatment involves surgically removing the extra skin during adolescence, *before* the problem can become serious.

Cramps and Dysmenorrhea: What Does The Pill Have to Do With Them?

Mary is a longtime patient with a sweet sixteen-year-old, Emily, whom I delivered. I can remember the moment I handed Emily to her mother, as those are the kinds of moments etched in my mind. Aside from having had the luxury of being a stay at home mom, Mary is your classic Helicopter Mother. This visit with her and Emily was a long time coming as Mary had been prepping me about how she wanted Emily to be my patient so that I could "guide Emily into womanhood." Emily was shy at first, explaining to me in front of her mother how she was just trying to do well in her classes and how she was too shy to talk to boys. I asked her about her eating and exercising habits, and when I asked about her periods, she started to well up. She described "crazy cramps" that kept her home from school and prevented her from taking part in volleyball practice and games. "I think something's wrong with me. If my cramps are this bad, does it mean that I won't be able to have babies when I'm older?" she asked. I reassured her that cramps are often a rite of passage for many women as puberty takes hold. I told her that I knew it didn't seem like much of a welcome, but that's what it was. Fortunately, I could put Emily on a low dose birth control pill to control her debilitating cramps. With that done, Emily was able to take part in all the activities that typical teenagers ought to be doing.

Oral Contraception (Good for the Tween V)

That medical boon to women, known simply as "the pill," is still the most popular method of birth control in the U.S.— although, perhaps not popular enough, since fifty percent of pregnancies in the country are unplanned. That said, there are more urban legends and myths about the safety and side effects of this oral contraceptive than any medication I know. In addition to its effectiveness in preventing pregnancy, the pill can help with a whole host of other ailments.

What can the pill do?

* Prevent pregnancy
* Lighten periods
* Regulate periods
* Control painful cramping
* Control irregular and heavy periods
* Control acne (*Wow, yes indeed!*)
* Balance hormone levels
* Treat symptoms associated with PMS
* Protect against ovarian cancer

And (drum roll, please) it is covered by most insurance plans!

To be fair, some women do experience *side effects* from the pill. Most notably, these include irregular bleeding, nausea, breast tenderness, bloating, and headaches. Of course, the pill *does not protect against sexually transmitted infections*, so condom use is a MUST! Also, you cannot take the pill if you have high blood pressure, a history of blood clots or strokes, or if you're a smoker older than 35 with migraine headaches.

But the most **debunked myths** about the pill go something like this:

* *But I'm going to gain weight on the pill!* I will tell you that study after study shows weight gain NOT to be a side effect of the pill. Most women start the pill in adolescence or when they head off to college, which IS a time when young women tend to gain weight. Unfortunately, the pill has borne the blame.
* *The pill will make me infertile!* Nope. No evidence to support this.
* *The pill will give me breast cancer and other types of cancers!* Again, there is no evidence to show that the pill significantly increases breast cancer risk, or the risk of any other type of cancer. In fact, the pill gives protection against ovarian, uterine, and colorectal cancers.
* *But I have to take a break from the pill if I've been on it a long time!* No medical reason to support this.

As you can see, there are many health benefits to oral contraception, in addition to its consistent efficiency as birth control! For most women, the benefits seem to outweigh the risks.

New Kid On the Block

"Breast tenderness, bloating, weight gain, emotionally crazy, on edge, a raging b*tch, or just not feeling right" are some of the common complaints associated with the birth control pill, which is the #1 prescribed medication used for contraception.

Birth control is simply a way of life and the easiest and most cost effective method has always been "the pill," but times are changing.

The intrauterine device, better know as the IUD, has been around a long time, but for many it's the "new kid" on the block since improvements on its construction have made it safe for women of all ages. The IUD, a small, flexible plastic device that fits snugly inside the uterus, is now considered to be an effective, safe, and long-term contraception alternative. Almost all women, including teenagers, are now candidates for the IUD.

In a recent Committee Opinion on adolescents and Long Acting Reversible Contraception (LARCs), the American College of Obstetricians and Gynecologists (ACOG) recommends the IUD as a "first-line" option for all women of reproductive age.

The Skylar IUD, which is smaller in size, may work best for those with a smaller uterine cavity like teens and women who have never been pregnant. We now know that IUDs are completely safe for all women regardless of whether they have been pregnant or not.

It is always best to discuss the risks and benefits associated with IUDs as a form of contraception. Studies show that the IUD has the "highest patient satisfaction" amongst contraception users. I would say the IUD is making a serious and purposeful comeback.

Adolescent Anxiety Is Real

Every year during her visits, Susanna speaks nonstop about anything and everything that comes to mind, including her daughter Emma. In the last couple of years I've learned about

Emma's struggle with depression and weed use, so I had at least a partial picture of who Emma was by the time Susanna brought her in for her first gynecological exam. I hadn't expected the very (too) thin, wan, angelic-looking 15-year-old seated beside Susanna. Susanna tossed her hair and fidgeted with her jewelry as she spoke for Emma. After a few minutes of this, I asked her to wait in the waiting room so that I could get to know Emma myself. Emma spoke softly and directly when I asked her about her period, cramps, eating and exercising choices. I learned that Emma's periods were erratic and often lasted two weeks at a time. I explained what I was doing as first I checked her thyroid gland, where I found a couple nonthreatening nodules (that were ultimately confirmed by a radiologist). Then I gave her a breast exam and finished with an external pelvic, which is when I noticed all too familiar cut marks on her inner thighs. I asked her what the cuts meant— even though I know that cutting is often a cry from girls who believe themselves unlovable—and after a long pause she started to cry. "I'm ready to get help...please," she told me.

Sometimes a visit to the gynecologist may uncover *other issues*. In fact, as per the U.S. Preventive Services Task Force, it is highly recommended doctors screen adolescents 12-18 for major *depressive disorders*, as eight percent of this country's adolescents experience an episode of major depression in a given year. Early diagnosis by someone trained in recognizing depressive disorders lends itself to early treatment and improvement of symptoms.

One in five adolescents have a **mental health disorder**— the most common being depression and anxiety—yet only half of those teens actually receive help. Oftentimes it's because depressed kids are not the ones likely to open up to their parents; rather they demand privacy as they try to navigate the world on their own and to figure out who they are. Also, adolescents tend to have less frequent healthcare visits than adults.

Problems common in this age group include bullying, body insecurities, divorce, drug, alcohol and tobacco use and abuse, self-injury (cutting), sexual identity and sexual pressures, to name a few.

Self-injury, which involves intentional cutting or burning of one's own skin, may very well go unnoticed by a parent—as in the case of Emma—since the areas cut tend to be hidden by clothing (a popular hiding place seems to be the inner thighs). Girls and young women are more prone to this than boys, and they often resort to this behavior in order to express themselves instead of finding a healthy way to cope with conflict. The pain of cutting skin serves as an emotional release. Fortunately, a visit to the gynecologist *exposed* the scars from Emma's cutting, but that was just the beginning for her. Psychological intervention will be needed to fully understand the cause of the behavior.

I believe that we gynecologists can be the gatekeepers for the mental health of our young women patients. We can help discern between typical tween anxiety and more urgent mental health concerns that may necessitate professional help. As I say this I realize that for most adolescent girls, *everything* feels urgent. I totally understand.

Role of the Healthcare Provider

Adolescents are generally a healthy group, but because their decision-making skills are still developing, their choices may be more impulsive or reckless, putting them at risk for certain health problems. Primarily, their health risks are related to their behavioral choices, not medical illness. During the initial contact between an adolescent and her healthcare provider, it's imperative the provider begins to develop a rapport based on *trust*. In order for this to happen, the environment must be one in which *confidentiality* is stressed, so that the adolescent may feel comfortable and unembarrassed in asking difficult questions during each and every visit. Confidentiality simply means that the patient has protection of privileged and private information discussed with the healthcare provider and their staff. It also means that the healthcare provider has legal discretion in knowing what should be kept as privileged and what can be shared with the parents.

Consider your daughter's healthcare provider to be an important teacher, one that will help to educate your daughter as the doctor–patient relationship grows. Topics of discussion should include age-appropriate information on female body development, body image, self-confidence, weight management, immunizations (including HPV), contraception, and prevention of STIs.

Regarding a pelvic examination, the American College of Obstetrics and Gynecology recommends one only be performed on patients younger than 21 if a medical history necessitates it. For instance, in the case of painful urination and/or abnormal vaginal discharge or odor, a vaginal culture might be taken.

Basic topics for discussion between your healthcare provider and your teen:

* Menstrual history
* Importance of starting breast self-exams
* Eating a healthy diet
* Daily physical activity

* Seat belt use
* Helmet use when biking, skateboarding, snowboarding, or skiing
* Bullying—identifying and avoiding it

Throughout the years, other issues may present themselves. Future visits may address behavioral problems and disease such as:

* Alcohol and substance abuse
* Sexually transmitted infections
* Condoms and birth control
* Depression and anxiety
* Pregnancy
* Eating disorders
* Tobacco use and Vaping
* Suicide
* Violence

The first complete and comprehensive gynecologic visit for an adolescent sets the stage for positive and informative dialogues that can help promote healthy alternatives. It's a time to empower our daughters in their sexual health and identity. It's a time that I'm especially grateful to be a part of.

When I sit across from a tween or young woman in my office and look into her eyes, I always feel the impulse to wrap my arms around her and say, "You need to take control of your body in every way. Don't be afraid to ask uncomfortable questions!" I want to tell these patients to learn about the hormonal changes that will wreak havoc with their teen years. I want to tell them not to be afraid to learn about and explore their bodies. Certainly, I want to implore them to make sure that their first sexual experience is with someone who cares about them as much as they care about that person. *She-ology* was especially written to arm Tweens with the key medical facts necessary to keep them safe, knowledgeable and healthy.

Unfortunately, adolescents still face the ongoing challenges of gender discrimination, which includes discrimination in education. I would like to see healthcare providers be on the short list of those who positively affect these young women. The tween and adolescent years are a time to question everything, especially when it comes to one's own body and health. Find a healthcare provider that your daughter (or niece or granddaughter) can connect with—it may not be *your* gynecologist, and that's okay.

One more thing: If my vagina revolution goes as planned, the owner of an adolescent V will not grow up to earn 78 cents to a man's dollar.

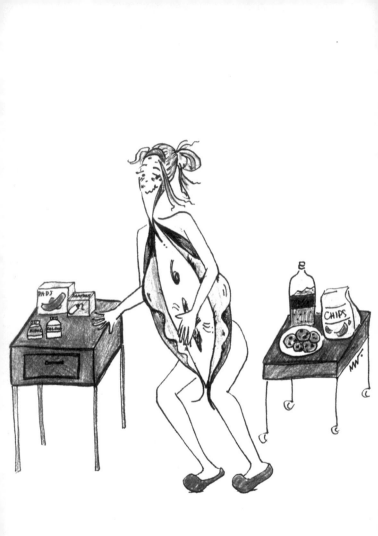

CHAPTER 3

hormonal

66 I am the ultimate multi-tasker, simply by necessity. My life runs in 10th gear most of the time, and around awards season it kicks into 11th. My priorities are my daughter, husband, family, and my work. As soon as my head leaves the pillow in the morning—5 a.m. most days—I am off and running.

The most joyful moments of my day are caring for my daughter, Alexandra, whom Dr. Sherry delivered when I was thirty-nine. There are no words to describe the overwhelming love and joy I felt when Dr. Sherry handed my beautiful little miracle to me just seconds after giving birth.

The most important job I've ever had is that of "Alexandra's mom." It is also the most difficult and rewarding job. What I want is to be the best mom possible to my little munchkin, which means that my husband, Jon, and I work as a team to manage our crazy lives and to give Alexandra all the love and energy we can summon each and every day.

She-ology

Nothing in my life is scripted unless I am working as the co-host of *The Insider*, and even that requires ad-libbing. I have been blessed to have a fun and exciting career in journalism, as a talk show host, lifestyle expert, and even as an actress. Anyone who knows me from my early days as a seventeen-year-old on MTV through my time on *The View*, *E!*, *Home and Family*, and *The Insider*, knows I speak the truth, which, in hindsight, sometimes works against my better judgment. Though, I'd like to think I have been able to give the younger generation perspective, no matter the subject matter.

Very few things can sway me from my daily routine, but those particular things are often beyond my control. Case in point: The week before my period I want to send in a SWAT team to put a stop to my PMS arsenal of symptoms which include bloating, water retention, and weight gain! During that premenstrual week my body is overtaken and transformed by hormones that take no prisoners. Honestly, they make my normal life a bit of a living hell! Going up a full bra cup size might sound like a good thing, but, unfortunately, not when your breasts are so sore that they make you want to cry. Imagine trying to do the red carpet at the Oscars, bloated with five extra pounds of water weight in a Zuhair Murad gown that was formerly perfectly fitted days before. Interviewing Leonardo DiCaprio, Matthew McConaughey, or George Clooney is a dream come true unless I'm sucking in my body within two inches of my life thanks to water retention.

PMS is truly my nemesis, but Dr. Sherry has given me a lifestyle treatment plan that has helped put a stop to this debilitating phenomenon. My counterattack on my hormones involves drinking a lot of water—two liters a day—taking calcium, magnesium and eating only fresh fruits, vegetables, and a high protein diet ten days before my period. I exercise every day, limit my sugar, salt and caffeine intake, avoid my favorite Japanese restaurant (soy sauce is the devil—even low sodium), and I don't drink any alcohol. I also eat foods that help

eliminate that awful bloating feeling altogether—cucumbers, asparagus and green tea, especially. Thankfully, this works every time; I love
you, Dr. Sherry. You have restored my sanity and my waistline!

—Debbie Matenopoulos TV Host

Seventeen-year-old Leanne, a senior at Santa Monica High,
loved playing the saxophone in her award-winning high
school band. It was, in fact, the thing that made high school
bearable. Though she first had her period at twelve, Leanne
had yet to have regular periods. In fact, it was a year between
her first two periods. Although she'd made peace with being
heavier than her friends, she was completely embarrassed
by her increased facial, chest, and upper thigh hair growth,
seemingly a result of hitting puberty. As she spoke of her
embarrassment and discomfort, her eyes welled up with tears.
She said she was so distressed that if it weren't for band, she
would ask to be homeschooled.

There's still a lot for us to learn about how hormones
work and what can be done when they are out of whack. Even
though hormones are the chemical messengers of our bodies,
coordinating everything from growth to metabolism and
fertility, the thing we women most associate with hormones
are the crazy mood swings, followed closely by the fatigue,
irritability, and anger (among a whole host of other mental,
physical, and emotional changes) that hormonal imbalances
may bring. As far as the vagina itself is concerned, from the
time a woman first experiences menstruation until the time
she stops menstruating, the menstrual cycle plays a role in the
appearance of the vagina as well as the hormonal imbalances

that can lead to cysts and conditions such as **PCOS**—the condition I imagined was plaguing Leanne.

Polycystic Ovarian Syndrome (PCOS)

Most of us have imagined how accommodating it would be to menstruate only once or twice a year. Sounds like a dream, but for the women who only have a period a few times a year, there is a good chance that the cause is a hormonal imbalance—not a dream situation. With monthly periods comes a feeling of emotional and physical balance, a suggestion that your body is hormonally in sync. When the balance is off, the cause may be a medical condition that can be disruptive to your normal routine, if not downright debilitating.

Polycystic ovarian syndrome is a medical condition that affects five to ten percent of women. It's thought that five million women in the U.S. suffer the symptoms of PCOS, which are brought on by an imbalance of estrogen and testosterone. These symptoms may include any combination of the following:

* Irregular periods—meaning that periods can be infrequent, heavy, and unpredictable
* Excess hair growth on the face, chest, abdomen, and upper thighs. This particular medical condition is called hirsutism.
* Obesity
* Oily skin
* Acne
* Infertility—Irregular periods mean irregular ovulation, so getting pregnant may prove difficult
* Multiple small ovarian cysts

* Depression and anxiety
* Male-pattern baldness or thinning hair

At the extreme of this condition, PCOS can lead to diabetes, heart disease, and cancer of the uterus.

As with many ailments, no one knows the cause of PCOS. What *is* known is that PCOS brings about an increase in hormones called *androgens*, along with a resistance to another hormone called *insulin*. High androgen levels, mainly testosterone, cause oily skin, acne, and unwanted hair growth. Because the hormone insulin controls the sugar (glucose) levels in our blood, higher levels of insulin cause you to feel hungrier than usual, which can lead to weight gain and obesity.

If you have irregular periods and notice hair growth in unusual places, please see your healthcare provider. A **diagnosis** of PCOS is made primarily on a physical exam coupled with a medical history. Blood work and a pelvic ultrasound will help in determining a diagnosis.

Treatment for PCOS

Since there is no cure for PCOS, treatment depends on the particular symptoms that you are experiencing and the degree of disruption you're feeling in your daily life. Don't be silently embarrassed by any of these symptoms—believe me, I don't think mustaches on women are going to be de rigueur for a while. Meanwhile, here are some of the symptoms along with their treatments:

* **Irregular periods:** Hormones, including the birth control pill or progesterone, are typically used to regulate the irregular and troublesome periods caused by PCOS. Long-acting, reversible contraceptives

(also known as LARCs), which include Depo-Provera, Norplant arm implants and intrauterine devices (IUDs), are frequently used to control erratic bleeding. Not only are these methods safe, they're convenient, effective, and they double as birth control methods. Depo-Provera, an injection given every three months, is an especially good option in relieving long and heavy periods.

* **Hirsutism (excessive hair growth):** The medication Spironolactone, often used to treat high blood pressure, is used to help control excessive hair growth, as is the birth control pill. Alternately, electrolysis and laser hair removal are non-medical ways to rid oneself of excess hair, although for best results, I would suggest a combination of medication *and* laser hair removal. My young patient Leanne found success for her excessive hair growth using Spironolactone, birth control, and laser hair removal over a nine-month period. Vaniqa, an FDA-approved prescription cream, is also helpful in removing facial hair.

* **Infertility:** Since women with PCOS do not regularly ovulate, getting pregnant can be tricky. Among the numerous medications to regulate ovulation, Metformin and Clomid are the most commonly prescribed. Seeing an infertility specialist is also an important step in making a pregnancy possible, since IVF is often necessary for a successful pregnancy in women suffering from PCOS.

* **Obesity:** Many women with PCOS tend to be overweight or obese and have a difficult time losing any weight. Not only is this frustrating, it can lead to

isolation and depression, especially in teenagers. A visit with a nutritionist is often the best approach to making successful food choices and achieving weight loss. In controlling your weight, you'll find that you may also control your irregular periods, excess hair growth, and acne.

* **Acne:** A dermatologist may be your best friend in combatting severe acne. Proactiv, a popular brand of skincare and acne treatment, works well, as my own kids can attest. Anti-androgens (medication which decreases testosterone) such as spironolactone can help reduce acne (as well as hair growth).

* **Long-Term Health Concerns:** Women with PCOS are more prone to serious medical conditions such as diabetes, heart attacks, high blood pressure, high cholesterol, depression, anxiety, endometrial cancer, and sleep apnea, which is why it's best to employ a knowledgeable team of experts, including a gynecologist and nutritionist.

PMS: <u>P</u>lease <u>M</u>ake it <u>S</u>top!

It's probably safe to say that we've all experienced (or continue to experience) the physical and emotional craziness that accompanies the week or two before a period. We're familiar with that three- to five-pound water retention, the short fuse, the cravings for all things sweet and salty (for me it was Kit Kats and Kung Pao Chicken), and the urge to sob watching Sarah McLachlan narrate ASPCA commercials featuring homeless and abandoned dogs. For some, premenstrual symptoms are only slightly noticeable, but for others the symptoms are debilitating, affecting school, work, relationships and life in general—it may seem as if you've being cast in a role for two weeks, 24/7, that *doesn't feel at all like yourself.* When symptoms are *that* severe, we are talking about **Premenstrual Syndrome (PMS)**, which typically encompasses emotional changes such as drastic mood swings, depression, crying spells, irritability, and anxiety. Physically, PMS symptoms include bloating, breast tenderness, weight gain, food cravings, and acne. A perfect storm which can lead even the sanest woman to feel as though she's become victim to an *Invasion of the Body Snatchers.*

The first thing to understand is why these changes happen in order to figure out a way to combat the symptoms of PMS. Fortunately, the majority of symptoms caused by PMS *can* be treated with diet, exercise, and the avoidance of certain key foods. The irony being that most women suffering from PMS seek immediate comfort from their symptoms in all these wrong foods!

Why Are We So Hungry Before Our Periods?

It's thought that the production and cyclical nature of the sex hormones estrogen and progesterone have a strong effect on appetite. Researchers have pointed to the increase of progesterone production the week or so before a period, which is responsible for binge eating. See, it *not* your fault! Estrogen, on the other hand, which acts as an appetite suppressant, peaks before ovulation and drops in the time before your period, adding a double whammy to your inability to fight those damn cravings. But don't despair. There is a way to eat in order to help your resolve as well as to resist those cravings.

* FOODS TO LIMIT OR AVOID: dairy, salt, sugar, caffeine, alcohol, Chinese food, and any other especially salty foods.
* Do drink as much water as possible, ideally two to three liters a day.
* Do supplement your diet with vitamins such as calcium, vitamins E & D, thiamine, magnesium, and omega-3 fish oil.
* Do eat healthy foods such as fresh fruits and veggies, protein-rich fish and chicken, and complex carbohydrates such as whole grains and brown rice.
* Do eat foods that are natural diuretics such as celery, cucumbers, watermelon, tomatoes, asparagus, lemon juice, garlic, melon, and lettuce. Doing this will greatly help reduce bloating and swelling *any* time of the month.
* Do reach for the green tea as a comforting beverage. It's a great natural diuretic and easier on the system than coffee.
* Do consider the herbal supplements dandelion, ginger, parsley, hawthorn and juniper, all of which help alleviate water retention.

Aside from adjusting your food, liquid, and supplement intake, there are other ways to treat the symptoms of PMS, no matter the severity.

* **Exercise.** I know it's the last thing you want to consider when you're overwhelmed by PMS symptoms, but it really does help. Regular exercise four to six times a week, for a minimum of thirty minutes a session is a must.

* **Acupuncture, Yoga, and Mindfulness.** These practices can help in controlling the mood changes and other emotional effects of PMS.
* **Medications.** Non-steroidal anti-inflammatory medicines such as Advil and Motrin can help with cramps.
* **Oral contraception.** "The Pill" can help control your hormones, cramps and acne.

For those of you who have tried all or some combination of the aforementioned but are still finding that there's no relief in sight, other methods may be needed to get you through the intense symptoms of PMS.

If you're wondering: When do I decide that my depression and/or mood swings are bad enough to try something else? The answer is that if your emotional state is preventing you from your regular daily activities and it's causing you to lose sleep and/or feel helpless, then you may need an anti-depressant or anti-anxiety medication. Certainly the emotional symptoms of PMS are well documented, but extreme episodes of symptoms such as anxiety can cause panic attacks, manifesting in heart palpitations, chest pain, dizziness, and shortness of breath. In this case, a diagnosis of **premenstrual dysphoric disorder (PMD)** may be made, and medication treating depression and anxiety can be prescribed. Fortunately, I have been successful in treating PMD and its debilitating monthly symptoms with a low dose anti-depressant (Prozac 10mg daily) and an oral contraceptive. I might add that it also doesn't hurt to swear off Chinese Food during the second half of one's menstrual cycle. Fight that salt craving if you can!

If you find yourself Pretty Much Suffering the majority of each month, help is available. Discuss your symptoms with your healthcare provider. Don't let half your life be disrupted by your menstrual cycle. There are treatments, and there's one that can be tailored specifically for your personal needs.

At forty-seven, Angelina is still the coolest girl on the block, which makes sense because she owns and operates the trendiest, most popular hair salon in Venice. Her bright fluorescent highlights make me want to experiment with my own hair, but then I would have to have her same effortless and carefree style. An avowed health nut, Angelina pretty much only eats what she grows in her backyard. When I walked into the exam room during her last visit, the first thing she said was, "Oh, thank God you walked in at just this moment, so you can see this wave of sweat. It hits me out of the blue all through the day!" Sure enough, her cheeks were bright red and sweat was beading around her upper lip and brow. Although she was having irregular periods, her blood tests came back as "normal" (meaning that she was not officially in menopause). But clearly, something hormonal was afoot.

Perimenopause

By the age of forty-five or so, there's a good chance you already considered how perimenopause would affect you. There's no accident that this period of hormonal disruption has been referred to for years as "the change." You've most likely wondered: *How will "the change" change me?*

It's different for everyone, but the constant questions I hear are: Will I have crazy uncontrollable bleeding for weeks on end? Will drenching sweats come on when least expected? Will sex become painful and sexual intimacy a thing of the past? To you all I say *hold on there*. First let's talk about what exactly happens in perimenopause.

Perimenopause happens when your ovaries cease to function consistently, thereby upsetting your normal hormonal rhythm. This hormonal change usually happens within a couple years of menopause, but for some it can happen much earlier. The erratic and disruptive symptoms of perimenopause tend, however, to mark the beginning of menopause. Every decade brings about some emotional and physical change, but for women, the decade of one's forties may pack the biggest punches of all. Between the typical forty-something anxieties of shifting relationships (divorce and dealings with hormonal or college-bound teens), self-esteem issues, job challenges and other midlife stresses, one's forties are challenging enough *without* the hormonal upheaval. In your forties, it's not just life's stresses that are affecting you emotionally and physically; it's "the change," the symptoms of which include, unfortunately:

* Irregular, erratic, and heavy periods
* Night sweats and hot flashes
* Mood swings with depression and anxiety
* Short term memory loss and trouble focusing
* Low sex drive (libido)

In order to be certain that you are, indeed, hitting up against perimenopause and not some other disease or disorder that may resemble it, such as PMS, thyroid disorder, depression, or early Alzheimer's, it's important to check in with your healthcare provider. A thorough medical history should be taken, along with a blood panel and a pelvic ultrasound in order to complete the final diagnosis. If the aforementioned medical conditions have been ruled out, then perimenopause is most likely the explanation for the symptoms such that Angelina described.

Treatment and Tips for Perimenopause

There are many different symptoms of perimenopause, and each may be treated differently.

* **Heavy and irregular periods:** The best treatment for this problem tends to be with hormones. Low dose oral contraception is at the top of the list as a way to control periods. Experiment with different pills in order to find the one with the least side effects. Other means of treatment include: cyclic progesterone, IUD with progesterone (Mirena or Sklya), Hormone Replacement Therapy (HRT), and non-hormonal alternatives such as acupressure and herbal therapy.

* **Hot flashes:** Dressing in layers and staying in cool temperature are the first steps in dealing with these flashes. Air conditioning is your friend! Plan ahead. Bring a cooler with ice to put to your hands or feet in. If you know that hot beverages, spicy foods, red wine and hot climates bring on hot flashes, avoid them (if possible). Herbal remedies may include black cohosh and other traditional Chinese medicine. Also, acupressure may help with mild hot flashes.

* **Mood swings:** Antidepressants are effective in controlling depression, anxiety, and panic attacks. A therapist may also give added support. And, of course, exercise, the elixir to all. When you exercise there's a natural release of mood-boosting endorphins and serotonin, the "feel good" hormones that your body can naturally produce.

* **Low sex drive (libido):** Testosterone therapy may be helpful for low libido. For help with a dry vagina,

vaginal lubricants such as KY and extra virgin coconut oil are a good and cheap investment. Sometimes, once you gain control of the annoying hot flashes, irregular bleeding and emotional distress of perimenopause, sexual interest is regained and your libido is rescued.

* **Aches and pains:** Acupuncture, an ancient Chinese treatment for maintaining health and vitality by balancing energy flow, works for many medical conditions. For women especially, headaches, lower back pain, menstrual cramps, and nausea may be helped through acupuncture. Even though the studies are not conclusive, hot flashes and heart palpitations may improve with acupuncture treatment. The believers are devout and many. This simple, ancient treatment can work well without causing side effects.

Perimenopause can be a challenging and confusing time in a woman's life. The good news is that the symptoms of this hormonal havoc are, for the most part, temporary—which means that they can last one to eight years, depending upon your body's reaction to your ovaries shutting down the production of estrogen. During this period life starts to move in slow motion and it seems like the hormonal upheaval will never end. Be aware that there are helpful remedies and sensible solutions. It's always best to follow up with your healthcare provider so you don't feel as though you are going crazy!

Menopause...

....The notorious, the musical (yes, it's still playing in Vegas), and for many, the hormonal nightmare. In the chapter **Mature**

46

Hormonal V

V, I get into the details of menopause, how it effects our lives, our physical and emotional well-being, and our vaginas. Briefly though, menopause is truly the final curtain call for the ovaries and their ability to produce estrogen and other sex hormones. But don't despair.

As was true regarding perimenopause, women in their forties and fifties just don't need another life stressor, but there's no avoiding the reality of menopause. The hormonal imbalance starts to peak between the ages of 45 and 55, bringing a host of emotional and physical changes. But as challenging as this time can be, it can also be exciting as it's the start of a new chapter of life.

By educating yourself on what is normal and what is not you will be better equipped to navigate your hormonal hurdles. Talk to your women friends to see what they're going through. Open up the menopause conversation and share your experiences (and symptoms), many of which will be overlapping with your peers. You'll find that not only are you not alone, other women in your menopause position are willing to lend a sympathetic ear.

My closest women friends and I have a running pool (that we began before any of us hit menopause). We bet who would be the first of our group of six to go into menopause and who would be the last! The woman who guessed which of us would be first and last wins a day of pampering at Heaven Massage and dinner at Blue Plate Oysterette! If anything, talking about how menopause is affecting us helps us to cope with the day-to-day vagaries. I encourage you to keep a dialogue going with a friend or group of friends with whom you feel comfortable, and maintain a connection with your healthcare provider as they will be able to help you make decisions about dealing with your changing self, whether it's through therapy, herbs, medication, etc.

The Hormonal V need not drive you mad! Find the right lifestyle changes and treatment options and keep the conversation open. You are not alone in this journey. Some of the best women I know are in menopause!

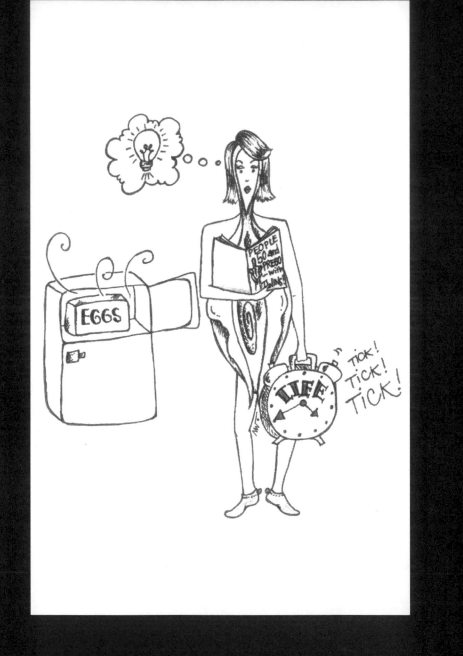

CHAPTER 4

baby maker

66 When I moved here, to Los Angeles, in my early thirties, I was told that for a woman to survive in this town she needed three things: a plastic surgeon, a shrink, and *a good gynecologist.* I was lucky enough to find a great one in Dr. Sherry.

Annual check-ups at her office felt less like appointments and more like getting together with a good girlfriend. We'd talk about work, relationships, boobs, and sex. Then one day, Dr. Sherry decided it was time we had "the talk." She asked if I had considered freezing my eggs.

I was around thirty-five at the time, and the thought sent a shiver down my spine. *Was I really getting past my prime for pregnancy?* After all, I was healthy, Botox had ironed out the first signs of wrinkles, and I was confident that Mr. Right was right around the corner. Plus, we were having this conversation more than ten years ago, when egg freezing was still considered experimental by the FDA. But Dr. Sherry was ahead of her time. She looked to the future, and she knew egg freezing was going to be the answer for hard-working women like me, who, for whatever reason, put pregnancy on pause.

But instead of freezing my eggs I decided just to chill. I went to yoga, grabbed a soy latte, and in the blink of an eye five more years went by. I turned forty. By that time my biological clock was ticking so loudly it was keeping me up at night.

Then one evening I met a tall, handsome man—he may not have been Mr. Right, but he was certainly Mr. Right Now—and we found we had one important thing in common: we both wanted to have a kid. So, first came our love, we skipped the marriage, and I started working right away to have the baby in the baby carriage.

Sure, I was pushing the pregnancy envelope, but this was Hollywood and everyone was doing it. Dozens of celebrities my age were on the covers of magazines with their newborn babies. *If it could happen to them, why not me?*

I had a million questions so I went looking for answers. After all, I'm a television reporter. It's what I do. And I quickly discovered women were not getting the whole story.

Getting pregnant after forty isn't impossible, but it's really, really difficult. By the time you hit your forties—statistically speaking—your eggs are mostly scrambled. Some of them are completely fried. Sure, there are some good eggs still left in you, but finding a perfect one is tricky. In vitro fertilization improves your odds, but it's expensive and it doesn't come with a money-back guarantee. (This is about the time a little voice in your head replays the conversation you had a decade prior with Dr. Sherry about freezing your own eggs.) Like many women, I warmed up to the idea w-a-a-ay too late.

So how are the rich and famous doing it? If you want the honest truth, they spend hundreds of thousands of dollars on fertility treatments. They freeze (and I'm not talking Botox) and they use donor eggs. For some reason, they don't talk about it—which I find ironic, considering celebrities openly discuss every other detail of their lives.

Here's the headline I want these lovely ladies to hear: Your celebrity diet, your skincare routine, or your favorite color of nail polish isn't nearly as interesting as the path you took to get pregnant.

Now, I'm not the most famous person to get pregnant at 45, but I do hold a microphone here in L.A., and I decided that if the celebrity moms weren't going to share their stories I would tell mine. So I proudly reported on TV news that I was pregnant, and I shared the fact that it was made possible because I decided to use a donor egg.

My pregnancy wasn't perfect. My ankles swelled and my Mr. Right proved to be all wrong, but one of my best friends never left my side—and, boy, did she deliver! Dr. Sherry was the first person to hold my beautiful baby boy, and I can't think of a better welcome to the world.

—**Wendy Burch** Emmy Award-Winning Reporter & Anchor

In my line of work, I have the immense joy of delivering babies, and though I've delivered hundreds of them in my decades as an OB-GYN, I'm still awed by their entrance into the world. I'm also acutely aware of the effort and planning and consideration that go with making the decision to have a baby.

For most couples, planning a pregnancy is simple: you have sex and—*voila!*—pregnancy. Unfortunately, that is not the case for many other couples or for single, 35-plus women with excessively *loud* biological clocks—for some over-forty women, the sound of those clocks is truly deafening. The couples and singles in these situations want to know what options and strategies are available. How soon must a woman plan for pregnancy? Can we push back the clock and make forty the new thirty—as countless TV shows, films, and magazine articles would like us to believe possible?

From fertility to birth, there are certain facts and figures that can't be argued, but there is also much hope—and technology—that I will do my best to disseminate for you. Ready, set—hold off on that layette just for the moment...

After years of fertility consultations and procedures, Wendy (yes, the Wendy who introduced this chapter) used a donor egg to complete her family. At forty-seven she gave birth to her son, Brady, and she's been on Cloud Nine ever since. When Wendy decided in her forties that she wanted a child, it was a moot case that I *did* ask her in her late thirties if she wanted to do any "family planning." As with many successful career-minded women, she thought she had all the time in the world.

All The Time in the World

File this under Believe It or Not: At twenty weeks a female fetus has six to seven million eggs, the most a female will have in her entire lifetime! Talk about the winds of time; from twenty weeks on it's all downhill, egg-wise. By the time a woman is about thirty-seven, she has only about 25,000 eggs left.

Fifty percent of pregnancies in the U.S. are unplanned, with most of those *unplanned* pregnancies occurring in women in their twenties, during the time that fertility peaks (usually between the ages of twenty and twenty-four). The other fifty percent of pregnancies are usually planned around careers, economic capabilities or constraints, or finding the right partner. For these reason (and others) motherhood is often delayed. Those remaining eggs? Well, they're waiting for no one, even though chances are that if you're having a baby beyond the age of thirty-five, you've waited for all the right reasons! And the truth is that when you've *chosen* to be pregnant, you are more mentally and physically in control of the process and more likely to make healthy choices in preparation of becoming a parent.

It used to be that the magic taking-off point for pregnancy worries was after age thirty-five. At thirty-four you were likely to be handed a "concerns for the older mother" brochure at your OB-GYN—*Older Mother? Who, me?*—but the American College of Obstetricians and Gynecologists now warns that "women's ability to have babies decreases gradually but significantly beginning around age 32, and then goes down more rapidly after age 37." After thirty-seven fertility declines at an increasingly lightening pace, so that by the time a woman is between forty and forty-five her fertility has decreased by as much as ninety-five percent, which leads us to...

The Fertility Conversation

When I first started out as an OB-GYN, the rule was to start having the F-talk (fertility conversation) with women at around age 35, but now the recommendation is to start that dialogue much sooner. Unfortunately, your healthcare provider may not think of starting the conversation, and not necessarily out of indifference. In today's busy, overburdened medical system, family planning is not always a priority. Ideally, the time to start counseling a woman about family planning is in her early thirties, but if pregnancy isn't an immediate issue there are usually other things that a woman may be concerned about, thereby putting the "planning" talk on a back burner. The problem is not only that women between the ages of 37 and 45 have a challenging time getting pregnant; they are also more likely to miscarry—the miscarriage rate being about fifty percent by age forty.

Don't count solely on your healthcare provider to bring up the fertility conversation; educate yourself about your prospects and make a special visit just to review your fertility plans, even if you don't have a partner. Being your own best healthcare advocate is especially important in the family planning arena.

Georgina is one ambitious Type-A 33-year-old attorney. I envied her dedication and drive. Despite her 60–70 hour-a-week schedule working in a large downtown Los Angeles law firm, she found the time to stay abreast of all the latest NPR news and the best Netflix documentaries. I did, however, worry about how exhausted she was on her annual exams—which she scheduled like clockwork. During a recent visit she'd fallen asleep on the exam table as she waited for me. I almost didn't want to wake her for her pelvic exam because she looked so uncharacteristically peaceful! But her eyes opened and the first words out of her mouth were, "I am already worrying about my ability to have a family! Listen, I haven't had a serious boyfriend in years and I don't see one on the horizon. Tell me about what I need to do to freeze my eggs." I have to say I was a little relieved to hear that Georgina had finally given the subject some thought.

Family Planning at the Techno Level

Egg freezing. Egg storing. It's the thing that gives women of all ages hope to use their own genetic pool to make a baby... sometime in the future. In 1986, the process of freezing (thereby storing) a woman's eggs was just entering infancy. The marginal success rate in defrosting frozen eggs made the process seem more experimental of an option than a viable one for family planning. Today, however, with better techniques and higher rates of success, egg freezing has changed the way that women traditionally chart their family planning.

A recent study found that the most common reason for a woman to freeze her eggs was a "lack of a current partner and not only to pursue career advancement." The Guttmacher Institute, a prominent reproductive health think tank, stated that "controlling family timing and size can be a key to unlocking opportunities for economic success, education, and equality" for women. They also found that this form of contraception "will help increase women's earning power" and ultimately "narrow the gender pay gap." That is surely a lot of positive reasoning in favor of egg freezing as an option to preserve fertility! It used to be that family planning meant the use of birth control—and the discussion of what types of birth control—to prevent pregnancy, but now egg freezing has become an entirely new type of planning for the future.

The time is in your early thirties to have a heart-to-heart with *yourself* and ask the following questions: How many children do I want? Am I willing to get pregnant without having a partner? How important is it to have my own biological child? You don't ever want to look back when it's too late and say to yourself: I wish I had been proactive in planning for my family.

Let's consider that you're now wanting to take this proactive stance. Current guidelines recommend that a healthy woman younger than 31, with a normal ovarian reserve—a properly timed blood test called AMH (anti-mullerian hormone) will give you this information—should evaluate her reserve every one to three years, since the best candidates for egg freezing are women between the ages of 31 and 38 who are delaying pregnancy by at least two years. I have noticed a trend in women in their twenties initiating the conversation and I have no problem supporting their family planning dreams. If you are a healthy woman older than 38 do not wait to meet with a fertility doctor and consider freezing your eggs. Women older than forty are still candidates for freezing, but their success rates in having a baby are less than ten percent. For those younger women, the success rate of a live birth with either frozen eggs or frozen embryos is forty to fifty percent.

This ultimate family planning policy of egg freezing is definitely catching on, and I'm thrilled to be part of the conversation around it.

Costs of Egg Freezing

At this point the cost of egg freezing often separates those who think about the process versus those who can actually afford to do it. One cycle of egg freezing can cost around ten thousand dollars, and, often, two cycles are needed to have a healthy egg account. Fortunately, companies like Facebook and Apple are at the forefront of embracing and protecting a woman's choice to delay motherhood. They are championing their career-driven women employees by supporting them in the family-planning department, which translates into including such support in health insurance benefits. It is my hope that routine preventative care for women will include fertility screening starting at age thirty.

Egg Quality and Quantity

I don't want to beat a dead horse here, but there's no way around this fact: The older you are, the fewer eggs you have, and the less likely that those eggs are viable. IVF is, indeed, a technological miracle, but it CANNOT make a forty-year-old produce more eggs, or make those eggs of better quality. Most infertility doctors will not (and should not!) even consider performing an IVF cycle on a woman 44 or older since the success rate is a mere one to two percent.

Ovarian reserve (egg health) is the term used in reference to how fertile a woman is compared to other women of the same age. In other words, not all eggs of, say, a 37-year-old woman are equal. The AMH (anti-mullerian hormone) blood test can help define the health of your eggs and can be taken any day during your menstrual cycle. This test helps to determine how many eggs are available and how healthy those eggs are regardless of your age. It's a simple test to help women in their early thirties know where they are individually in their reproductive life. The result may push you towards freezing your eggs, starting a family, or having the luxury of waiting for future use. AMH also predicts how many eggs a woman is likely to make in a single egg-freezing cycle. Ideally, a woman would produce fifteen to twenty healthy eggs in one cycle, which is an easier feat to accomplish for women in their early thirties. For those who aren't high egg producers, two or three cycles may be necessary in order to secure a couple dozen eggs. An FSH (follicle stimulating hormone) drawn on Day 2 or 3 of the cycle is also a helpful predictor to determine the health of your eggs.

Ultrasound is another means of checking on egg health. During the beginning of your menstrual cycle, usually around Day 2 or 3, an ultrasound can determine how many small follicles containing eggs are in each ovary. The medical term for this is an "antral follicle count." Clearly, the greater number of early egg follicles, the better—ideally, six or seven follicles per ovary suggest healthy eggs are brewing.

If you've begun your research on fertility, chances are that you want to know your egg health or ovarian reserve. You probably want to know how your eggs compare to those of other women your age. That's a good start in taking part of your own family planning, and with these inexpensive tests you will find out whether you need to see an infertility specialist sooner or later.

Game Changer: The Donor Egg

Even if you are older than 44 and unable to count on your eggs to give you a biological baby, you most likely can count on your uterus to *carry* a pregnancy. Dr. Hal Danzer, a well-known infertility doctor in Beverly Hills, reminds patients that if they cannot conceive with their own eggs, "donor eggs are the best chance of success," especially if a woman is over 44 (typically, healthy egg donors are under the age of 25). The truth is that regardless of biological age, almost any woman can become pregnant using a young and healthy donor egg. Most often a donor egg is the last resort.

After Wendy had exhausted all hope of having her own biological baby, she decided that a donor egg would fulfill her dream of giving birth to her own child. Wendy went online to My Egg Bank, a trusted egg bank in Atlanta, Georgia, where she was able to review detailed profiles of young and healthy, anonymous egg donors. At My Egg Bank she was able to look not only at the baby photos of potential donors, but profiles of their personalities. "Almost like ordering on Amazon Prime," Wendy told me. A five-foot-ten, 22-year-old third-year college student studying to be a journalist turned out to be Wendy's ideal donor. Wendy ordered the eggs online. Her doctor, the aforementioned Dr. Danzer, received the eggs two weeks later, which were then fertilized with the sperm of Wendy's fiancé, ultimately creating a healthy embryo. Two weeks later one embryo was implanted into Wendy's uterus. As you already know, the rest is history.

Women who use a young, healthy donor egg have a forty- to fifty-percent chance of getting pregnant during the first IVF cycle, which are good odds when you're determined to have a family—although most infertility doctors will not do IVF using a donor egg on women older than 53 due to the medical complications associated with this age group. If you go the donor egg route, you have the peace of mind in knowing that the egg is legally yours—no chance of losing parental rights once the baby is born.

On a personal note: When I was in my early thirties, a dear friend and patient of mine asked if I would be her egg donor. She'd recently remarried and desperately wanted to have a baby with her new husband. She was in her early forties at the time and had suffered a couple miscarriages and failed IVF cycles. How could I not help? Interestingly enough, what initially was meant to be a favor to a friend wound up being a heartening and exciting personal experience. My friend and her husband had a beautiful set of twin boys, whom I delivered via C-section. I've never felt any maternal connection to the twins; rather, I *have* felt an extra degree of tenderness and love in knowing that I was able to help complete my friend's family. It gives me tremendous joy to watch these beautiful and talented young men growing up. I would do it all over.

She-ology

"I'm an open book, which is probably a good thing, since I live much of my life on a reality TV show. It also helps that I say what I think and I have an opinion on most things, including the belief that God works in mysterious ways—S/He certainly does! I do believe that finding Dr. Sherry Ross after my second miscarriage was a lifesaver. But let me back up just a bit.

Two years ago, with a baby in tow, I started as the star of my own reality show on OWN, Oprah's network. Early into the show, surprise-surprise, I became pregnant, so the producers and I thought, "Great! We'll work it into the show and follow the entire pregnancy." Sadly, I miscarried, but the show went on and the cameras continued rolling. The whole emotional experience became part of season one.

Cut to the beginning of season two. They say lightening never strikes the same place twice, but that was before *Livin' Lozada*. Once again, I became pregnant early in the season, and then, once again, in a nearly identical manner, I lost the baby, which is when Dr. Sherry came into my life. She has pretty much been holding my hand ever since. Of course, I have Carl, my husband-to-be, at my side, but my other "partner" in my trials has been Dr. Sherry.

Soon after season two finished, I got pregnant again—yes, Carl and I desperately wanted a baby—but when I went to see Dr. Sherry she seemed intuitively to know that it would probably not be a successful pregnancy. Unfortunately, she was correct, but she also had a solution in mind. She suggested IVF treatments. She told me not to feel guilty for having done anything "wrong" during my pregnancies—which is how many women mistakenly feel after an unsuccessful term—and that, clearly, I was fertile, but my mature (I only just turned forty!) eggs were probably the cause of my miscarriages. I struggled with the decision. I thought: Did my miscarriages mean that I wasn't meant to have another child, or was I being tested? Was I supposed to persevere and go after what I wanted, as I'd always done? I certainly didn't want to live with the guilt of not having at least tried to get pregnant again, even if it meant using an unconventional method.

Be on the lookout, because I'm trying my first cycle of IVF before you can say, "Stay tuned until next season!" And, most fortunately, thanks to Dr. Sherry, I've a plan and all the information I need, so despite my fear of big needles (ouch), I am proceeding full speed ahead. 99

—**Evelyn Lozada** Reality TV Personality

In Particular...Women Older Than Forty

I know, it sounds like the title of a new sitcom about cougars and mothers or mothers who are cougars, right? And by the time of this printing there probably will be one, but women in this particular group are increasingly looking to get pregnant. The truth is that I'm the first to appreciate a woman who takes good enough care of her body to pass for younger than her actual years. I do appreciate the workouts and commitments to healthy choices and the mindful living that goes into looking and feeling younger, but the reality is that women older than forty have a five percent chance of getting pregnant. You may have spent the last forty years doing everything in your power to slow the aging clock, and you may still fit into your perfect size 6 jeans from high school, but your eggs do not reap the benefits of that healthy living. They don't ignore the aging process the way the rest of your body may (for a time, at least).

I know this is a hard pill to swallow for many women past forty, especially for those who are misinformed, which is why it's so important to understand your own egg health and quantity before you hit forty *if you're planning on having a family.*

Plans for that family, however in the future they may be, need to be made early on.

Barring that, if you're still intent on pregnancy, I encourage you to be proactive and meet with an infertility specialist as soon as possible in order to optimize each monthly ovulation.

After 45...

Good, you're still with me. And here's the skinny on getting pregnant without help after forty-five: Women older than forty-five have a *less than one percent* chance of getting pregnant each month of trying. I know, you may have picked up a *People Magazine* or tuned into *Entertainment Tonight* just to be met with the headlines of another celebrity woman past the age of forty-four giving birth...to twins no less! This news can be incredibly misleading since it does not include statistics on such pregnancies, or include the extensive time and cost of employing *fertility magic*. Donor eggs are usually the secret ingredients in this celebrity pregnancy mix if the woman is older than forty-four, especially if she is having twins!

But **Janet Jackson** is having a kid at fifty! Well, sure, I heard the news as well. Janet is finally taking time off from her career to take care of her long-awaited pregnancy. What the news doesn't mention is that Janet would have had a less than one percent chance of getting pregnant using her "elderly" fifty-year-old eggs. Maybe that is what happened. Maybe she did win the genetics lottery, but I suspect that, realistically, Janet either froze her younger eggs or used a donor egg. Whatever the means, don't be misled into thinking that there's no rush—*if Janet can get pregnant at fifty, then so can I!* It's true; you can *be* pregnant, as long as you embrace reproductive flexibility. Don't take the pregnancy of a fifty-year-old woman at face value; rather, use the circumstances to spur your education on how such a miracle is possible. And plan ahead!

Other celebrities who probably had a little help in their reproductive journeys include Geena Davis, who had twins at forty-eight, Halle Barry, who had a second child at forty-seven, Kelly Preston, pregnant at forty-eight, Marcia Cross, twins at forty-five, Beverly D'Angelo, twins at forty-nine, Cheryl Tiegs, twins at fifty-two, and Holly Hunter, twins at forty-seven. Laura Linney was forty-nine when she gave birth and Jane Seymour had twins at forty-five. I do understand the reproductive process is a very intimate thing and many women do not want to share the details of their own particular journeys, but what I would like to have happen is simply a conversation. Meaning, the next time you read (or see) that some Hollywood beauty is pregnant at forty-five, especially with twins, consider she used her own frozen eggs or donor eggs. That is the seed (literally) of the conversation, rather than thinking to yourself, "Gee, if those women had babies with their own eggs, then so can I."

As savvy and informed as my patient Wendy was, she still thought, at forty-something, that she had time to use her own eggs to have a baby. After jumping through all the infertility hoops and spending thousands of dollars to no effect, she finally decided to select a donor egg. Once that decision was made, the rest was easy.

Older Moms: Medical Risks

Unlike women in their twenties, women older than 35 are more at risk for genetic and chromosomal abnormalities, hypertension of pregnancy, diabetes, preterm labor, and cesarean sections. The risk of these complications is twenty to thirty percent higher for women past 35 and fifty percent higher for women older than forty.

When certain other variables are also at play, the risk may be higher, which is the reason why a *surrogate* may be used. A surrogate is a woman hired to carry one or more embryos to a full term baby. Through IVF an embryo is transferred into the surrogate's uterus. The embryo may be the result of the patient's egg, a donor egg, or the surrogate's egg combined with the partner's sperm or a donor sperm. There is any number of combinations resulting in an embryo, which is then implanted into a carefully chosen surrogate.

For some women, carrying a pregnancy is impossible. It may be due to problems such as large uterine fibroids, endometriosis, hysterectomy, or an unrelated complication such as heart disease, which would make pregnancy extremely dangerous. Gay men also use surrogacy to have a child.

To illustrate a happy ending in which a surrogate was used, I'll let **Kimberly Quaid** tell her story.

I always knew one thing was certain, I wanted to have babies and be a mother. When I was married I tried desperately to get pregnant, but for reasons beyond my control it didn't happen the old fashioned way, so I turned to a method that seemed promising in the wake of my particular fertility problems, intrauterine insemination, which involved placing sperm inside my uterus and multiple IVF attempts. I thought: Mission accomplished, pregnancy done, birth on the horizon.

In all, I attempted in vitro seven times over the course of four years, and in all that time the only conclusion my fertility doctors could draw was that my infertility remained "unexplained." Unexplained. It sounds so ordinary and harmless, but believe me I nearly lost my mind as I became more insistent on continuing after each failure. It became debilitating as well as agonizingly depressing. Even so, I couldn't imagine my journey to parenthood was over. I became more determined than ever. As if on cue, a neighbor of mine mentioned surrogacy. I barely remembered ever hearing the word before, but it suddenly was a mantra for hope. Believe me, it was scary, but the idea of not having children was even scarier. My family and my fertility support team thought it was a good idea and encouraged me to choose a surrogate, which I did—using the agency recommended by my neighbor. My surrogate was what is called a gestational carrier, which meant that she would carry my egg fertilized with my husband's sperm. In fact, she became pregnant on the first try with two of my fertilized eggs.

It seems so bizarre to recall this time in my life in such a clinical manner, but to try and recall just a fraction of the emotions I went through would prevent me from ever telling this story. That is to say, what happened after my first try at surrogacy was beyond devastating. My surrogate miscarried, first one baby, on Thanksgiving, and then the other, on Christmas.

I had two eggs left, so in the final attempt my surrogate got pregnant with twins. My surrogate's pregnancy was uneventful, and I was over the moon. Again, it's odd, but I can barely say the rest of the story aloud without choking up. Seven and a half months into the pregnancy, my surrogate was in a terrible auto accident. Her car was totaled, but, miraculously, she and the unborn twins were fine. Preterm labor followed. The twins were born healthy and are now amazing 3rd graders. 99

—Kimberly Quaid Mother of Thomas and Zoe

One thing you need to know about surrogacy is that it is costly. The $50,000–$80,000 price tag includes the fertility process along with the reproductive agency and attorney fees, but there are many avenues you can take in finding a surrogate. You may want to ask a family member, a friend, or a reputable surrogacy agency. However you proceed, know that surrogacy can be an exciting, successful option.

Lifestyles of the Baby Makers

For most of us, everything feels just a wee bit (or a lot) more difficult as we age, and pregnancy is hardly the exception. It's challenging at any age to find the energy to get through the day, get enough sleep, and exercise regularly, and even more so for the pregnant woman who is carrying and nourishing a whole other person within.

Your fertility is affected by many factors—genetics, age, diet, body weight, lifestyle, medical and contraceptive history, and stress. It's proven that stress leads to depression and anxiety, which can affect fertility, so in order to reduce stress it's important to manage it. Relaxation training, mindfulness, yoga, and acupressure are successful ways to battle the negative energy and help you towards and through pregnancy.

Alcohol, caffeine and smoking also affect fertility. Trying to conceive? Limit caffeine to one 12-oz. cup a day and quit alcohol and smoking altogether. Smoking not only affects your fertility, it increases your miscarriage rate. Over a long period of time, it also leads to poor egg quality and early menopause.

Obesity—which refers to a BMI measure of more than thirty percent—also causes hormonal disruption, which can lead to infertility.

A **male partner** who is planning on supplying his own genetics to the mix might wind up with abnormal sperm production if he has a tendency to smoke marijuana on a regular basis, or if he uses Propecia for hair loss. Both marijuana and Propecia have been known to affect sperm production. In fact, infertility is not just caused by factors in a woman's health. **Male infertility** affects forty percent of infertile couples; so make certain that your partner is paying extra attention to his own personal lifestyle habits. After all, he's playing on a *team*.

Prenatal vitamins are an important addition prior to conception since they contain extra amounts of folic acid, which is necessary in the prevention of neural tube defects and autism. Adequate levels of this mineral are recommended at least four weeks before conception and at least eight weeks after the start of pregnancy in order to be most effective. Research suggests that taking folic acid pre-conception reduces the incidence of neural tube defects by fifty to sixty percent, and new studies show that women who take folic acid prior to conception and in early pregnancy may have a reduced chance of having a child born with autism and severe language delay. Take your vitamins!

Baby Makers, I would hope that at this point you know how important the care and maintenance of your vagina is, but I would also hope you educate yourselves on how age and lifestyle affect fertility. Talk to your gynecologist or meet with an infertility specialist to determine what's ahead in order to secure future fertility. If you know you want your own biological baby, but are not ready to commit to becoming pregnant, consider freezing your eggs. Ideally, this is best to do before you're 35, but it can be done up to age 42.

Routinely, I question my thirty-something patients not only about the regularity of their periods or their safe-sex practices, I ask them about their future plans in the baby department. It's an important question, and an even more important conversation. Take the time to ask yourself about your own fertility plans, and then bring up the subject with a trusted healthcare provider. Your wakeup call shouldn't be a deafening biological clock sounding tomorrow "It's time!" Your wakeup call is now, in these words.

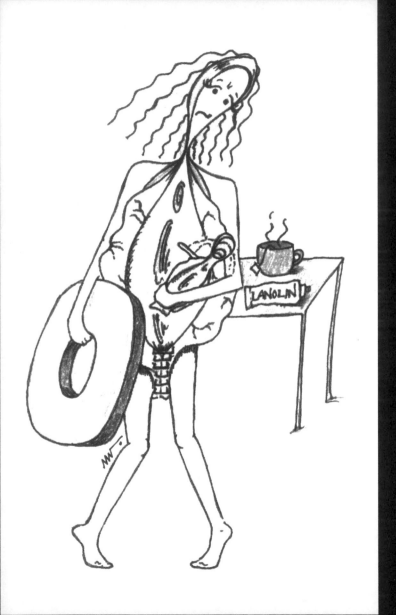

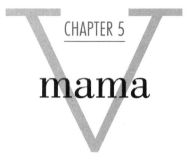

CHAPTER 5

mama

"All I have ever known for sure was that I wanted to be a mother. From the time I was old enough to hold a child, I knew I wanted children of my own.

My journey to becoming a mom was fraught with countless disappointments and repeated heartbreak, but after seven attempts at IVF and one miscarriage, I finally became pregnant. Because of the miscarriage and a past surgery addressing severe cervical dysplasia, I was told I had a compromised cervix and was therefore an "at-risk pregnancy."

Thankfully, I had a surprisingly pleasant and uneventful pregnancy devoid of morning sickness. I even did yoga until a week before delivery. I loved being pregnant, and except for feeling tired—which has always been a given for me due to my tendency to have countless things on my plate—I felt terrific.

She-ology

When my water broke I went to the hospital, where I was put on Pitocin. After 24 hours in labor I was rushed into the ER for an emergency C-section because my baby's umbilical cord was wrapped around her in three places. Eventually the hospital team rescued her from the warzone that had become my uterus, and she emerged healthy and unscathed. I, however, was not. My uterus had herniated and I had lost a great deal of blood. The team needed to decide whether or not I would need a blood transfusion, a hysterectomy, or both. Ironically my compromised cervix was just fine, although my exposed organs gave the delivery room the look of a gory picnic.

Having decided on a more conservative "wait and see" approach, my doctor reassembled said organs inside my body and a 24-hour wait began. Back in my hospital room, my baby was brought to me to breastfeed, but I couldn't recognize her as someone I knew. I felt disconnected, as if I were under water. In fact, I looked around the crowded room at my husband and mother, in-laws, stepsister, and oldest friend, and I hardly recognized any of them. My father had died three weeks prior, but I expected him to walk in and greet his granddaughter—and namesake. I felt a million miles away from the smiling, celebratory faces around me. I was watched closely throughout the night, and by morning I was told that I was "all good to go." No hysterectomy or transfusion needed.

The next few weeks were some of the worst of my life. I was terrified for no discernable reason and I felt no connection to my child. My husband was gutted by my inexplicable despair and the darkness that seemed to have engulfed our lives. We had no idea what was happening. Eventually, after confiding my feelings to my doctor, he diagnosed me as having PPD (postpartum depression).

I began a multi-level treatment plan, and then, slowly, we all emerged from the shadows.

Mama V

This "fourth trimester" of a pregnancy, which is aptly referred to as "postpartum hormonal chaos," can be a devastating period of sadness, confusion, shame, and fear.

The terrifying thing about PPD, aside from its devastating effect on all involved, is its lack of discrimination. Because hormones have a mind of their own, PPD can occur with your first child and not the second, or rear its ugly head only with the third. It can even sneak up on you two years after a child is born.

Surprisingly however, when my desire arose to have a second child I honestly had no reservations. The reason being that I was *informed*. I was determined not to go through the same trauma the second time around. I would not be victimized by the insidious nature of PPD. What eliminated my fear was a thoughtful and deliberate plan of action for my particular circumstances. Dr. Sherry and I analyzed my previous condition and we devised a plan that would fortify and protect me from the potential onset of PPD. In my case, the plan involved a monitored dose of medication in the third trimester, a scheduled C-section, and a close emotional and biochemical monitoring of my wellbeing after childbirth.

The result of such vigilance was a stress-free pregnancy and a delivery the likes of something out of a Disney cartoon (if babies were delivered in Disney cartoons). More importantly, although the postpartum period was accompanied by the normal extremes of exhaustion, I maintained a true sense of wellbeing and even peace. I was balanced.

It is imperative for women to take the reins on their wombs! Take the necessary precautions prior to delivery and don't try to "power through" if, after delivery, something doesn't feel right. Being your own personal health advocate does not make you high maintenance; it makes you informed and in control.

Surround yourself with a support team, whether it is a therapist, obstetrician, nutritionist, acupuncturist, family member, or friend. And no matter how many people there are to cheer you on, take care of yourself. Exercise, a balanced diet, and a proactive stance during your entire pregnancy and into postpartum is essential. Ask questions, not just about your baby, but about yourself. In this chapter Dr. Sherry discusses topics that should be part of your normal conversation with your OB.

Be proactive. Think of your pregnancy as being for a lifetime, instead of just a few trimesters. All you are feeling and doing matters, and you are not alone. 🙶🙶

—**Brooke Shields** Actress, Entrepreneur, Spokesperson

You ever feel that there's one supermom doing everything right? Well, that's the feeling you'd have about Julie. She's the one who ought to be *giving* the free Whole Foods lectures on how to make natural, homemade baby foods, the one who knows which products are purest, and can give you the lowdown on everything organic, paleo, and sustainable. Of course, Julie also had the perfect pregnancy. I mean, do you know anyone who gained a textbook perfect 29.6 pounds total and breezed through a natural birth without any pain meds while suffering only a two-degree vaginal tear? Julie breastfed religiously from the start—before weaning her baby onto food from her backyard garden—and never had a complaint pregnant or postpartum, until her husband brought up the subject of sex. Ah, SEX, the new frontier in motherhood. Right to the point, Julie said to me, "My vagina is dry, sex is painful, and it's the LAST thing on my mind when my head hits the pillow, or anything resembling one! I can't even remember what my 'old' vagina feels like! Plus, my breasts are leaking all over the place. I am so not feeling in the mood, and forget about feeling SEXY. Is there anything I can do to at least make sex tolerable?"

Imagine: You've given birth in a hospital and you're ready to take your tiny new person home. Probably you've a bag of departing gifts that includes the hospital magazine, diapers, formula, coupons for more diapers and more formula, and a disposable pair of granny panties big enough to draw a full-sized bullseye on. I've always thought, how is it possible that no one thinks to hand a new mom a *manual* of sorts? At the very least there ought to be better communication between the new mother and her healthcare provider, especially at this start of all hormonal hell breaking loose.

Like Julie, you may feel as though someone has surreptitiously replaced your vagina with something alien. I'm here to tell you, hang on...

Help Is On the Way for Your Mama V

First off, there's a lot going on during this period, which I refer to as the "Fourth Trimester" of pregnancy. **Postpartum** is the least talked about time during the pregnancy cycle—chances are you may not be aware that it is *part of* that cycle. From the moment your baby is delivered, until the time that your body has completely recovered, you are postpartum, which is why the exact time for this period varies from woman to woman throughout the first year. If you've had a vaginal delivery, the vagina and **perineum** (the area between the vagina and anus) have literally and figuratively gone the distance and will take a considerable amount of time to heal. Pain and discomfort are common during this period.

The first week following a vaginal delivery is difficult for a variety of reasons, not the least of which is due to your hormonal transition. Your body is getting rid of the forty percent more blood and fluid volume that was needed during pregnancy. Can you even imagine a radical new diet that amps up weight loss in such a way? It would surely leave you exhausted, if not a little crazy.

Within the first forty-eight hours you start to have intense, pajama-drenching sweats, typically at nighttime. The reason for this is hormonal fluctuations that lower your estrogen levels while elevating your prolactin levels, (prolactin being the hormone that stimulates milk production) which prepare your body for breastfeeding. Here's your chance to experience what a menopausal hot flash might feel like as this dramatic reduction of estrogen levels parallels the *menopausal experience*—more on that in the next chapter. Even if you choose not to breastfeed, your body will still undergo these symptoms (but on a lesser level) as your milk supply dries up, allowing your prolactin and estrogen levels to normalize.

Which leads us back to Julie, our perfect mom who is just looking for some "tolerable sex." Painful intercourse, clinically known as **dyspareunia** (which sounds remarkably like an exotic form of melancholy) is a common occurrence. At six weeks postpartum it's reported that fifty to sixty percent of women suffer from dyspareunia, and a third of women will continue to have symptoms three months after delivery.

Dyspareunia may be due to vaginal tears, episiotomy, damage to the pelvic floor muscles or, if you are **breastfeeding**, the hormonal effects of low estrogen. We're seldom made aware that these low estrogen levels cause vaginal tissue to become thin, dry and pale, similar to the attributes of an atrophied vagina. It's no wonder that sex might be painful. In some cases it's almost like going back to sex after a twenty-year absence.

Imagine...or not! There's less blood flow to the vagina, resulting in a decrease in vaginal lubrication. Dryness, irritation, burning, itching, painful urination, painful intercourse... these are all common symptoms.

But I'm Breastfeeding! Isn't that Supposed to Help?

Yes, of course, but as wonderful as nursing is for your growing baby and for enhancing the bond between the two of you, it prolongs the pain (and suffering) of vaginal dryness, hormonal upheaval, and low sex drive. If you've had kids, you've been there. No one escapes, but time, understanding, and patience, along with some KY jelly and estrogen cream, can make the Mama V a little bit happier.

The C-Section vs. Vaginal Birth... Less Pain?

In regards to painful, post-pregnancy intercourse, when women who'd undergone vaginal deliveries were compared to women who had Caesarean Sections both groups were found to have the same discomforts. (No need to secretly envy your C-section sister whom you imagine has escaped all vagina angst.)

For those who deliver vaginally, depending upon whether or not you had an episiotomy or vaginal laceration, your ability to move freely can be limited and painful at first, making even the simplest of activities difficult. Trauma to the vagina can be significant—imagine a cantaloupe emerging from your vagina—for as miraculously elastic the vagina is, there's only so much stretching it can do before it tears. Realize that it can take up to four weeks just to heal your Mama V.

Soothing the Mama V

With time, the symptoms of pelvic pain and painful intercourse will improve, and interest in intimacy with your partner will do the same. Meanwhile, there *are* things you can do to soothe your (if not savage, at least *irritated*) V.

During those first few weeks following a vaginal delivery, helpful remedies may include sitz baths (simply, a warm water bath), ice packs, and lidocaine spray (a local anesthetic). For centuries women have been crafting solutions like freezing pads or diapers and placing them in mesh panties. But now, one of the most wonderful new remedies for the Mama V during these challenging weeks is the Mama Strut by Pelv-ice. The Mama Strut is a total pelvic support with highly adjustable multi-directional compression and ice/heat therapy to manage pelvic pain and swelling exactly where a new mama needs it. Woman using the Mama Strut not only have a whole lot less trauma after giving birth, they need fewer narcotics, have increased mobility, and experience better moods than women who suffer through without any help.

Later on, depending on the severity of the pain, some women choose to use vaginal estrogen cream two to three times a week to reduce the symptoms of vaginal atrophy. Over the counter vaginal lubricants, extra virgin coconut oil, and topical lidocaine can be used to ease the pain in intercourse— which is to say, help you to enjoy it once again. Be empowered to take control of your pain management and healing.

And then there's *sleep*, the *final frontier* for some. No doubt about it, **sleep** is good for every aspect of recovery.

Sleeping well at night or taking naps during the day will help you to maintain your sanity and patience, as well as give you the strength for all your new (and old) routines.

Speaking of old routines, resuming your **exercise** schedule will not only help you to lose your pregnancy weight, it also will give you more energy throughout the day. Which leads us to...

So When Can I Start Exercising?

How soon to resume your exercise regimen will vary according to your physical and mental condition, your regimen prior to and during your pregnancy, and, of course, your delivery experience. If you had a traumatic delivery and/or an episiotomy you may not be able to resume even the easiest exercises until three to four weeks postpartum. The sutures used in repairing an episiotomy typically dissolve within four weeks, so it's best not to overextend yourself during that time. If you begin a strenuous workout sooner than your body is able to handle, you'll set back your postpartum recovery. Be reasonable in your workout routine—you don't want to ride a bicycle or take a spinning class for at least six weeks following an episiotomy repair (you may even wince just thinking of it).

However, if you've had an uncomplicated delivery with minimal trauma to your perineum, you may start light exercise as soon as one week after delivery. Walking is an excellent transition into more advanced cardiovascular workouts, and it has the added benefit of clearing your head. Your joints are still *loose* during the first six weeks postpartum, so although you may feel that you can attempt a split for the first time since high school gym class, those loose joints can interfere with your coordination and balance. Start your exercise regimen slowly *and* with your healthcare provider's blessing. Until then, you can at least start those *Kegels*.

What About Those Kegels? My Girlfriends Say I Have to Do Them.

Your girlfriends are *correct*! Start those Kegels as soon after delivery as you remember to. Pregnancy and childbirth can weaken your pelvic floor muscles, resulting in uncomfortable pelvic pressure and unwanted leakage of urine (try sneezing without those muscles). Kegel exercises are a simple and effective way to strengthen those pelvic floor muscles, which support the uterus, bladder, and bowel. They can help delay or even prevent *pelvic organ prolapse* (protrusion of the pelvic organs into or through the vaginal canal) and other related symptoms.

Kegel exercises are easy and can be done anywhere, anytime, without anyone knowing you're doing them! First: Identify your *pelvic floor muscles*. The easiest way to do this? Next time you're urinating, try to stop the flow of urine midstream and hold it. Hold that contraction for three seconds, and then relax, allowing the flow of urine to continue. Repeat this a couple times and you will have successfully identified your Kegel muscles. If you're doing this correctly, you will feel your pelvic muscles squeezing your urethra and anus.

Once you've identified your pelvic floor muscles, you can perform your Kegels. This time, empty your bladder and then sit or lie down. Contract those muscles and hold for five seconds. Relax for five seconds. Repeat. Try doing this routine four or five times in a row. Work your way up to maintaining the contraction for ten seconds at a time, relaxing for ten seconds in between. Your mission (should you choose to accept): a minimum of three sets of 10–15 repetitions a day. These exercises will not only strengthen your pelvic floor muscles, they can also make sexual intercourse more enjoyable for you and your partner. Make those Kegels a permanent part of your daily routine.

Patience

It takes nine months to journey through pregnancy. Allow your body (and vagina!) the same nine months *postpartum* to return to normal. With time, the Mama V will recover!

Depression and the Mama V

At forty, Sarah was an educated, highly successful (and anxiety prone) CPA. She had all her eggs in a row—that is, except for the one she most wanted. She'd recently met Ben, the man of her dreams, who, thankfully, had passed muster with her mother—an important milestone in Sarah's life. Sarah could hardly wait to have a child. At forty-one, concerned about the quality of her "older" eggs, she and Ben opted to start IVF cycles. They went through three cycles before becoming pregnant, but then the thought of labor so paralyzed Sarah that she insisted on an elective Cesarean section. The delivery went without a hitch, but as soon as Ben showed his wife their new, sweet, baby Madeline, I could tell something was wrong. Sarah turned from her husband and newborn and asked Ben to take the baby away. She didn't seem compelled to bond with Madeline. Breastfeeding was so agonizing that she had to stop after fifteen days. Insomnia and prolonged crying jags prevented Sarah from giving Madeline even the most basic of care. Sarah returned to her pre-pregnancy therapist, who prescribed Wellbutrin in an attempt to get her back on track.

Meanwhile, Ben moved his mother in with the family in order to help care for the baby—that, in addition to a night nurse. Eventually, Sarah wound up at the UCLA Mental Health Center for further treatment.

The startling fact is that eighty percent of women get the baby blues to some extent. That's eighty percent of *all* women— Hollywood celebs like Hayden Panettiere and Gwyneth Paltrow, my favorite Trader Joe's manager, a successful type-A career gal like Sarah, and someone else who you probably know. Anyone can fall victim. It shouldn't take a postpartum woman drowning her three children in the family bathtub to wake up women (and their family and friends) to this common malady.

Once your baby is born, you may think: *Hey, I've done all the hard work already, the baby's fine, I should be fine!* You may wonder how it's possible that you could land right in the midst of a perfect storm. Like I've said, the postpartum period officially starts the minute the baby is born and continues for *at least* six weeks! You get a postpartum "pass," which gives you a one-year body (and mind) recovery period after the feat of childbirth, which you greatly deserve! The hospital and staff may have been superbly attentive throughout your childbirth experience, but that doesn't help you overcome the feeling that your hugely oversized abdomen will ever be the same. Everyone is quick to acknowledge (and commiserate with) your lack of sleep, but you're still trying to come to grips with the pain from pushing through your own personal ring of fire and wondering why no one's discussed your ridiculously sore nipples or the reality of your post-preggers body. Aside from all that, your to-do list as a new mom feels almost insurmountable. No matter how helpful your partner is, or how many family members, friends or hired helpers you have, there are things that only you can and want to accomplish.

It's a little overwhelming. Let's just start there. Two to three days after delivery, amidst all the wonder and joy (that everyone keeps reminding you of) you, as the new mom, may be feeling a little less than wonderful. Depression, anxiety, and frustration creep into the situation, manifesting in crying jags over seemingly "nothing." You may be unable to sleep, eat or think clearly, and you may be at a complete loss for how to care for your new "bundle of joy"—again with the "joy" factor. Unlike postpartum depression, which I'll talk about in a moment, the blues diminish within a couple weeks after delivery. The joy becomes apparent as your temporary blues dissolve.

Beyond the Blues

Postpartum Depression affects ten to fifteen percent of women, making all those feelings of anxiety and desperation debilitating to the point where you are unable to go about your daily routine, including caring for your baby.

The main symptoms of this kind of depression include severe mood swings, intense irritability and anxiety, panic attacks, overwhelming sadness, uncontrollable crying, loss of appetite, insomnia, feelings of inadequacy as a mom, and, to a greater extent, thoughts of harming yourself or your baby and notions of suicide. These symptoms can continue for months. For this reason, it's very important to acknowledge your feelings. Information about the prevalence of postpartum depression is finally readily available to healthcare professionals all over. Safe to say it no longer carries the stigma it once did.

What Variables Might Increase My Risk of Postpartum Depression?

* **History of Depression or other Mental Disorders:** If you've suffered from depression or some mental disorder before or during your pregnancy, not surprisingly there's a greater likelihood of you suffering from postpartum depression. If you have a history of postpartum depression, you also risk the same this time around.

* **Emotional Factors:** If your pregnancy is unplanned and/or you're feeling doubtful and insecure about having a baby, you are at a higher risk.

* **Fatigue:** Indeed, the "F" word. Prolonged fatigue after giving birth or having a C-section increases your risk of postpartum depression.

* **Lifestyle:** Having little or no support from a partner, family, or friends or being in the throes of a major move, a family tragedy, or illnesses are factors linked to postpartum depression.

* **Hormonal Changes:** These types of changes during pregnancy may trigger depression. The hormonal rollercoaster ride of pregnancy can reverberate in painful consequences after the ride is over.

* **Difficulties in Breast Feeding:** A study recently revealed that mothers who stopped breastfeeding due to pain or problems in nursing were more likely to develop postpartum depression than those moms who stopped breastfeeding for other reasons. Pain in breastfeeding, cracked nipples, breast infections, poor milk production, the inability of your infant to latch

on or suck—these are all factors linked to higher risks of depression. Let's acknowledge that it's a challenge to breastfeed, so if you choose to do so you need additional support. Don't hesitate to reach out for help!

What Do I Do Now?

The effect of hormonal chaos is a postpartum given, so it's sometimes difficult for you or a loved one to distinguish postpartum depression from the usual (and temporary) baby blues. However, if you *suspect* that you or a loved one may be suffering from this **treatable** condition, the first thing to do is contact your obstetrician or healthcare provider.

Treatment of Postpartum Depression

Once your medical provider has screened you for postpartum depression, your treatment may include a combination of drugs, including antidepressants and anti-anxiety medications, coupled with psychotherapy. Be patient—it can take three to four weeks for medications to start working, but they will help manage the symptoms of your depression.

Though extremely rare (occurring in less than 1% of women) postpartum psychosis may be the diagnosis. In these uncommon cases, the symptoms of postpartum depression are joined by hallucinations, delusions, paranoia, confusion, and attempts at harming yourself or your baby.

The Agony and the Ecstasy!

The exhilaration of holding your newborn for the first time can't be overstated, but it can be overshadowed by an unexpected flood of other feelings and emotions. For many, the birth of a baby triggers an emotional chaos that may spiral into something frightening and seemingly uncontrollable. The medical community understands that postpartum depression is a *complication* of giving birth, a treatable complication at that. Through medication, psychotherapy, and support, you will survive. Vital to that survival is open and honest communication with your partner and family. If you *or your loved one* experiences signs of depression and withdrawal, it's imperative to seek out help with a healthcare provider.

Know that with time and patience you will emerge from the dark tunnel of postpartum depression. In the interim, ask for help. Don't travel through that tunnel alone.

Lastly, while we're on the subject of asking for help, no matter whether your blues are manageable or debilitating, this postpartum period is the time when contact with your healthcare provider needs improvement. Insist on the communication that will help you to understand what the heck is happening to your body. Ironically, the hormonal changes postpartum are similar to those in menopause, yet I'll bet my best speculum that few healthcare providers make that correlation, at least not aloud to their patients. Educate yourself by asking the tough questions—describe what's going on with your body, your boobs, your mind, and your vagina. Say the words. Demand comprehensive answers. You and your Mama V deserve as much.

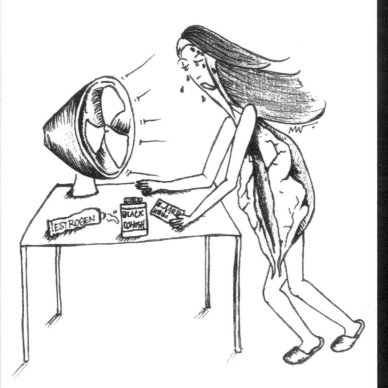

CHAPTER 6

mature

66 My forties were pretty much a blur. I gave birth to my twin sons at forty-five, and after breast-feeding for six months, my periods returned on an annoyingly irregular basis. Apparently I was in pre-menopause, right on the heels of pregnancy, birth, and breastfeeding—what a treat. I started natural estrogen and progesterone as soon as I could to control the symptoms, since I'd heard from my very vocal girlfriends just how horrible those symptoms might get. I'd already experienced a few hot flashes in bed that drove me to fling my legs out from under the covers in all crazy directions just to cool down. When dressing for the day, I'd wear layers so that I could strip them off easily. Hence, I became addicted to wearing decorative shawls!

There might have been more daytime hot flashes, but, frankly, I was too busy running after my twin toddlers to notice. Was the sweat dripping off my face due to chasing my boys in the park on a 98-degree day or the sign of another ill-timed hot flash? I'll never know.

Since menopause proved not to be the debilitating monster I'd been warned about, I didn't think I needed hormone replacement therapy. Truthfully I was worried about the increased risk of breast cancer, which I'd read was a factor in HRT. Since I'd been a ballet dancer, I did have the beginnings of osteoporosis, so I started on the bone-strengthening medications Actonel and Boniva instead of HRT.

In time, I started to experience an uncomfortable dryness and burning in my vagina—especially during sex—along with unintentional loss of urine (please, remember, I had given birth to four children!). Dr. Sherry knew exactly what to do. She started me on estrogen in the form of the Estring (an Estradiol vaginal string). Not only was it the easiest of solutions (it only needed to be changed every twelve weeks), it was a lifesaver for my dehydrated vagina!

Dr. Sherry and I have known each other for more than twenty years, since she came on set to do a "house call" for me when I was on the TV series *Dr. Quinn, Medicine Woman*. We hit it off from the start, and she has been my close friend and trusted doctor ever since. Dr. Sherry has always advocated for women and asked them to embrace their health care, and to not be afraid of asking tough questions— including those having to do with the Mature V—which is why, I imagine, she wrote *She-ology*.

I've always felt that humor was important in dealing with female health-related issues—a little humor, combined with open, honest discussions with a trusted doctor. I've been blessed to have such a doctor, one who is not only brilliant, but also encouraging, tactful, and skilled in getting me to open up about some very private issues. I'm not sure that would have been the case with a male doctor.

My Mature V, I'm happy to say, is perfectly functional and as content as I am in my life. Here's to health, love and happiness with your Mature V. 99

—Jane Seymour Actress & Artist

Mature V

At fifty-five, Janis had the energy, looks, and bounce in her step of someone twenty years younger. She'd come to see me with one of the most common concerns I hear from otherwise healthy women her age; after twenty-four years of enjoying sex (in this case, with her husband) she was having major pain and discomfort with intercourse. It initially seemed as though Janis had staved off the usual vaginal difficulties of menopause. After all, she'd gone into menopause three years earlier and, except for an occasional hot flash, didn't experience anything to disrupt her days or nights. She righteously maintained, "Menopause will not slow me down!" She added, "I will definitely not go on hormone replacement therapy no matter what! My friend went on HRT and got breast cancer six months later!" But lately Janis had been noticing pain, burning, and dryness with intercourse, making sex nearly impossible. She was understandably upset and told me, "I miss the intimacy and connection with my husband in bed. Please don't tell me that there is such a thing as **'old lady' vagina**! There must be something I can do!"

Just the Facts (Disclaimers and Myths), Ma'am

Whoa, first things first, and then we can cycle back to Janis' concern about the totally unscientific correlation between a mere *six-month cycle of HRT* and, bang, The Big C.

First, may I present the biggest change for the Mature V, The Big M—**Menopause**. In this chapter I hope to address the many, myriad questions that you may face with your Mature V—the emotional as well as the physical and psychological—so that you do not have to be sidelined as you enter this next, exciting chapter of your life.

Medically speaking, menopause is a *natural* condition in which your ovaries stop producing the estrogen that your body and vagina have, up until menopause, relied on. When estrogen production stops, so does your menstruation. Since the main function of estrogen is to support the development of the female body and the female secondary sexual characteristics, it only makes sense that when estrogen is gone, every part of our body that makes us female is affected, some worse than others.

Old Lady Vagina

Turn and face the strange... ch-ch-changes.

Well, yeah, you and I both know that Bowie wasn't necessarily talking about that particular strange change of menopause or shifting internal organs, but for me, the sentiment is the same.

My most recent strange was my [deep breath] atrophied vagina. Before that it was the unexpected detonation of early onset menopause. Oh, yeah, that's what those night sweats and my short temper were all about—well, maybe not the short temper; maybe that was genetically unavoidable. But anyway...

My atrophied V: that was my most humbling experience of late. There it was, yet another physical demarcation of time and life galloping on and my having to find a way to face the changes in my body with some humor and grace.

The beautiful thing is, I'm not alone. As I speak with my women friends—because, damn it, with kids and work and logistical nightmares I haven't yet found the time to actually *see* them—I realize that we are all reading from the same Mature V script, which seems to be some variation of: (To child) "Honey, I can't remember *everything* for you. I need a little help." (To spouse) "Not now, I'm too tired." (To self) "What the hell is happening to my vagina?"

Mature V

And what I've learned, aside from the fact that life in itself is a humbling experience, is that there are always challenges. The script changes somewhat, but the challenges remain, and I'm happy to report there are often solutions, as is the case concerning the Mature V.

Throughout the years, the compassion and knowledge of my OB-GYN, Dr. Sherry Ross, have had a profound effect on how I view myself and my changing body. Dr. Sherry has helped me address those changes by providing practical and creative solutions along with a necessary dose of humor (sometimes following a good cry on my part).

Our life "script" may sometimes call for us to fake our good cheer, our enthusiasm, or even our orgasms, but we don't have to fake the attention we pay to our precious bodies and selves. Please, read on, with the awareness that celebrating and attending to your Mature V can make all the difference in your enjoyment of life. And embrace those *ch ch changes*.

—LisaGay Hamilton Director & Actress

Fact: Yes, your vagina ages, just as you do. Disclaimer: Your vagina does not have to feel old. In fact, there are ways to keep it youthful and elastic. The menopausal vagina is a mature vagina and it can be treated in ways so that neither you nor your partner will suffer.

With the loss of estrogen to nourish and hydrate the vagina, the tissue becomes dry, pale, and dehydrated. The labia can become fused, and the vagina and clitoris may shrink. The medical term for this is vulvovaginal atrophy (VVA). As a result, intercourse, other forms of vaginal contact, and even walking and exercise can become painful if not impossible. Oftentimes these symptoms are accompanied by urination problems, such as an increase in urgency and frequency, but, as I mentioned, there are things that can be done to counter. VVL

Non-prescriptive remedies for VVA may be your first go-to. These include lubricants such as KY, gels, moisturizers, and oils, which can ease and minimize the discomforts of menopausal vagina. A great, natural, alternative lubricant is extra virgin coconut oil. In fact, I am almost 100 percent convinced that extra virgin coconut oil has singlehandedly saved the marriages (or romantic partnerships) of many of my patients. Take the oil testimonial of my patient Rachelle:

56-year-old Rachelle breezed through early menopause with only a couple years of hot flashes and insomnia, nothing that warranted medical treatment. Still, for the first time in seventeen years of marriage, she was not enjoying sex because of her excessively dry vagina. "My current lube is so not cutting it anymore," she told me. "Is sex just going to be painful from now on?!" I recommended she purchase a jar of extra virgin coconut oil, to which Rachelle responded, laughing, "What is extra virgin coconut oil NOT used for?!" Three weeks later, Rachelle called to say that she had taken my advice, and that she and her husband had a new lease on bedroom life. She even went above and beyond, using the oil on every square inch of skin. Apparently, the more the better.

Now, as wonderful as coconut oil is, it is not the answer for everyone. In the case of more severe menopausal symptoms **localized estrogen treatment** can help and even reverse the dry, painful condition of your vagina. **Oral Hormone Replacement Therapy** (**HRT**—more on this later) and **vaginal estrogen** are the two fastest treatments. **Osphena**, a relatively new non-estrogen prescriptive, is now available to help with vaginal symptoms related to low estrogen.

Vaginal estrogen comes in the form of weekly tablets, creams or a vaginal ring that you leave inside your vagina for twelve weeks. If you chose a prescription vaginal estrogen therapy you will not be exposed to the possible long-term risks associated with HRT. With vaginal therapy you ought to notice a reversal of symptoms in about three to four weeks. But wait, there's more...

On top of the personal pain and frustration, VVA is also extremely damaging to intimacy in a relationship since it can make intercourse impossible. Vaginal therapy is not only important for your physical health, it's important for your emotional health. It's important for your vagina, your partner, and the two of you as a couple. Male partners often feel guilty having sex with their partner knowing they are causing pain as a result of VVA. Women often want to avoid sex since they know it will be more painful then pleasurable. Having a conversation with your partner about your suffering vagina may be tough even if your communication is usually free and easy.

MYTH: If My Vagina Closes Up, My Sex Life Is Done Forever

Many women suffering from vaginal atrophy have usually not had regular vaginal penetration. That lack, combined with VVA, can result in a shrinking of the vaginal opening, which may be combatted with the use of a vaginal dilator. A survey found that 45% of women have never actually had an honest conversation about their vaginal dryness with their healthcare provider. They may have resigned themselves to sexual intercourse only once or twice a month or on "special occasions," giving the term "birthday sex" a whole, new despairing meaning.

To begin the process of opening up again, literally (and perhaps figuratively), vaginal dilators may be employed to stretch the vaginal opening. Usually the process involves use of a dilator for twenty to thirty minutes, three to five times weekly, gradually increasing the size, with the goal of making vaginal penetration easier on the tissue. Used in combination with weekly estrogen cream therapy, symptoms related to vaginal atrophy may be reversed, allowing painless (and, with luck, *enjoyable*) intercourse. As long as you're at it you might try soaking in an Aveeno bath for twenty to thirty minutes a day as a pampering addendum to treating vaginal skin as well as the skin over your entire body.

Alternatives to conventional dilators can be found not only at a local sex toy store in the form of dildos and vaginal vibrators, they're also at your local farmer's market, in the form of cucumbers or zucchini. If you do however choose a ubiquitous form of produce, make sure you use a condom on it to avoid unwelcome bacteria. A pea-size dollop of topical lidocaine applied to the entrance of the vagina also helps in avoiding pain when introducing anything into a sensitive vagina, be it vegetable or mechanical. **VVL**

Because some of my shyer and less adventurous patients don't know where to begin, I have gone online in my office with them in order to scroll through dildos on goodvibrations. com, a great, accommodating online sex store that caters to women. While we're perusing the endless array of toys, I ask these shyer patients of mine to try and approximate their husband or partner's "size." I tell them to decide on a color—*No, what color do you prefer?* I ask them to choose a special lube, to pick a vibrator. "What else?" I ask. "What else is on your wish list here?"

I'm glad to say that most of these patients report back with promising results after conventional vaginal therapy combined with a little fun (perhaps in the form of a classic purple dildo). Realize that when you enter menopause it's not just the vaginal pain and dryness that can ruin a perfect date night, it's the worry of vaginal collapse from infrequent intercourse. If you are having problems not only with dryness, but vaginal shrinkage and pain, please talk to your healthcare provider. Keep in mind that creative strategies are not only fun, but may be a necessity!

No Prescriptions, Hormones, or Medications Need Apply

Meet the Mona Lisa Touch Laser Treatment, the newest kid on the block to combat vaginal atrophy. An Italian built laser device, the FDA-approved Mona Lisa Touch Laser holds tremendous promise in treating a vagina that has been transformed in menopause. Once you've had a pelvic exam to assure that you are an appropriate candidate, a physician trained in the use of the Mona Lisa—which is actually, a small vaginal laser—inserts the device into the vagina during three 3-minute sessions, six weeks apart. Many women report positive changes after just the first 3-minute treatment, which involves removing the dried skin inside the vagina, thereby stimulating collagen production and allowing vaginal revival. The end result is a vagina makeover—a new lease on a vagina, if you will—with more elasticity and natural lubrication of the tissue inside the vagina. Although it may sound too good to be true, the results are proving to be a game-changer in the way vagina atrophy is being treated—without hormones—which is a relief to many women and their partners.

Mona Lisa is ideal for the woman who cannot take estrogen due to a personal or family history of breast cancer or for those who are unhappy with the side effects associated with HRT.

The success of the Mona Lisa Touch Laser is undeniable. Many satisfied customers are singing its praises, claiming that they are not only able to have *sex* again for the first time in ages, they are actually enjoying it. Seemingly, the most painful part of the procedure is the cost, which runs about $1000 a session and is most likely not covered by insurance.

Bottom line: Quality of life, especially in the bedroom, is incredibly important and should be a priority. VVA does not have to ruin you and your partner's sexual (or emotional) relationship. A vaginal preparation used two to three times weekly, at bedtime, can reverse any of the aforementioned disruptive symptoms associated with VVA without an increased risk of breast cancer and the side effects related to long-term hormone replacement therapy. Don't hesitate to discuss this common problem of VVA and its possible treatments with your healthcare professional. No more suffering in silence, please. **VVL**

Hot Flashes... Those Other Menopausal Symptoms

Rae Ellen, a 47-year-old high-powered executive lives her life in one gear—6th! A minute in her powerful presence is long enough to let you know you should not be fooled by her delicate, petite frame. When I hugged her on a recent visit, despite the comfortable cool of my office, I felt her face was dripping wet. She knew she'd "slimed me," as she called it, and then added, "Are these hot flashes supposed to be a fucking cosmic joke? My mother never experienced anything like this. Christ, it's only 10 a.m. and this is my seventh fucking flash. My head is about to explode. I had to get dressed twice this morning because I sweat through my favorite silk blouse after my morning latte!"

Seventy-five percent of women experience **hot flashes**, which are described as sudden bursts of heat in your face, neck and chest, causing you to sweat profusely. Hot flashes last three to six minutes, sometimes longer, and can affect your ability to sleep and function normally. The most intense hot flashes occur in the first two to three years of menopause, but some women have them into their eighties!

Non-Hormonal Remedies for, as Rae Ellen So Succinctly Put Them, "Those Fucking Flashes"

* Behavioral and lifestyle changes have been known to go a long way! One suggestion is to remember to always layer your clothing, that way you can easily pull off and on a layer as you feel a flash coming. An avoidance of alcohol, tobacco, caffeine, and spicy foods has been known to ease symptoms, also (don't laugh) try keeping a portable fan in your bag for a quick and easy cool down! In addition, a practice of relaxation, yoga, and mindfulness can go a long way in helping to control mild symptoms.
* Herbal remedies such as black cohosh, soy, and red clover may be helpful for mild hot flashes, although clinical trials did not find those herbs to be more effective than placebos.

* Acupuncture has had mixed reviews on the hot flash front. Since acupuncture has relatively no side effects if done correctly, I do believe it is worth trying. As with herbal remedies, it may even have a placebo effect.
* Brisdelle, better known as Paxil, is a low-dose anti-depressant that seems to help minimize hot flashes. Effexor and Prozac are other non-estrogen alternatives that have also been found to be helpful in treating hot flashes. I'm not suggesting that your vagina needs an antidepressant, although it and you may feel that way!

MYTH: Menopause Is Just a Phase

Here's the thing, menopause is the next chapter of your life, not a phase that you go in and out of like puberty. Many women believe that once the obvious and most common symptoms of menopause lessen—such as hot flashes, sweating, insomnia, depression, anxiety, apprehension, weight gain or loss, fatigue, poor concentration, memory loss, heart palpitations, exacerbation of migraines, and vaginal dryness—menopause is done. Not so; rather, it may be just the beginning of your new "normal." Yes, many of these symptoms do improve over time, but knowing that doesn't help when you're at the height of discomfort. All of these symptoms can disrupt the quality of life, but they can be lessened and, in some cases, eliminated with simple medication and lifestyle modifications.

Sex Drive: Where'd It Go, and When's It Coming Back?

When menopause strikes, the estrogen level plummets. For many, the **libido** (sex drive) follows suit. When your ovaries shut down during menopause, the production of estrogen *and* testosterone also shuts down, affecting your sex drive and your desire to be intimate. Frustrating and distressing sexual problems peak at midlife (45-64) for women—not a big surprise for most of us in this category. Low sex hormones plus vaginal dryness equals a decreased libido. What to do?

Testosterone cream may be helpful in this age group, but it's still considered "off-label," meaning it has not been a proven antidote for low sex drive (I've concluded that it has a 50/50 track record in the bedroom). Also it's important to be aware of the potential side effects of testosterone treatment, which include acne, facial hair growth, aggressive behavior, and voice changes. If you try this treatment, just be aware of its limitations.

And as long as we're on the subject of hormones, it's time to address the dynamic duo of estrogen and progesterone in **Hormone Replacement Therapy**, which is proven to help in combatting vaginal drying and improving low hormonal levels (and thus, low sex drive), and equally proven to polarize the members of any number of Friday night book clubs.

HRT...Let's Dive Into the Discussion

Ask ten of your girlfriends of a certain age how menopause is affecting them and you'll get ten different answers. Everyone has a different story to tell, and certainly *everyone* has their own take on the merits and demerits of HRT. Take my patient

Janis, who was certain, without any practical correlation, that six months of HRT was the cause of her friend's breast cancer.

The medical consensus on HRT, mainly estrogen, is that it's the most effective treatment for disruptive menopausal symptoms. In an overwhelming number of reliable medical studies, the benefits of HRT outweigh the risks, if the treatment is before the age of sixty or within ten years of menopause. Not only that, but HRT may also prevent osteoporosis related fractures. As pointed out earlier, lifestyle adjustments are, indeed, helpful in controlling the emotional changes associated with menopause, but HRT definitely has a place in treating depression and other mood changes.

If you're thinking of trying HRT, it doesn't matter whether you take it every day or cyclically (meaning that progesterone is taken every fourteen days to induce a period). You will not be at an increased risk of endometrial cancer or pre-cancer with either treatment regimen, however the current recommendation for HRT is to take estrogen-progesterone therapy every day if you have an intact uterus. Side effects, especially in the first six months, may include breast tenderness, bloating, and uterine bleeding.

So, after all is said and done, *is HRT safe?* It has been established that the major risks of hormone therapy are blood clots and breast cancer, with a slightly increased risk with combination estrogen-progesterone therapy, however the risk is *less than one additional case of breast cancer per thousand cases.* If you take only estrogen, you are not at an elevated risk.

With so much "pink" (read: breast cancer) information directed at us, the fact that one in three women will die from heart disease is often obscured. Of course, your risk of heart disease is dependent on your age, personal risk factors such as family and medical history, and lifestyle habits such as smoking, obesity and alcohol consumption, but did you know that estrogen protects against heart disease? Your risk of heart disease increases with your age and reduction in estrogen. If HRT is started within ten years of menopause, or before sixty, the risk of heart disease is minimal; therefore, the benefits outweigh the overall risks. In fact, women who go into premature or early ovarian failure may be started on estrogen therapy just to insure some heart protection.

Generally, I encourage women who have opted for HRT to try a lower dose after seven years, unless they find that their menopausal symptoms are uncontrollable. The ultimate goal over time is to be on the lowest possible dose of HRT. That said, there are women for whom HRT is not a good idea.

HRT should not be used by women with:

* Liver disease, history of deep venous thrombosis, or pulmonary embolism
* Known blood clotting disorder or thrombophilia
* Untreated hypertension
* History of breast cancer
* Women with high risk factors for breast cancer
* History of endometrial cancer
* Hypersensitivity to hormone therapy
* History of cardiac heart disease
* TIA (Transient Ischemic Attack)

The Biggest Myth of HRT

HRT will make me fat. Not. Look, weight gain in menopause is a reality for many of us, but it is not the HRT that will make you fat! Many women past the age of fifty and on HRT tend to blame their weight gains on the therapy, but that is not the cause. Plain and simple, as we age it is harder for us to lose weight. The hormonal upheaval of menopause tends to make weight gain in the usual places—abdomen, thighs, hips and buttocks—a common complaint. That upheaval, along with aging, genetics and lifestyle choices, makes losing weight all the more challenging. Some believe that you need to eat 200 to 300 less calories to maintain your current weight once you hit fifty, but the main focus for women should be on eating a healthy, well-balanced diet, regularly exercising, and limiting alcohol consumption.

Fact or Myth: Bioidentical Hormones Are Natural and Much Safer than HRT

At 54, Gretchen has logged a couple decades in search of the fountain of youth. Her husband of twenty years bestows upon her a generous allowance to do whatever necessary to keep her beauty as it was when they married—interestingly enough, Gretchen's doting husband is also twenty years her senior. Gretchen came to see me for a second opinion on the bioidentical hormones prescribed to her by an "Eastern" gynecologist, a "specialist" in bioidenticals. She had been taking 8 MG of Biest, a compounded estrogen formula, (now bear in mind that according to the largest national compounding pharmacies, 2.5 MG dose of Biest is the common transdermal estrogen preparation) and 100 MG progesterone twice a day for two years! She saw her doctor every three months for blood tests, ultrasounds of her uterine lining, and salivary testing of her estrogen levels. For several months she'd had irregular bleeding, but her doctor told her not to worry about it. She was in my office for the very reason that she couldn't stop worrying, so I performed an endometrial biopsy and found pre-cancer cells in her uterus.

Okay, as a teenager I loved the TV series *Three's Company* as much as the next person, but Suzanne Somers would not be my go-to gal on the merits of bioidentical hormones. First of all, the FDA, an independent group that regulates and tests for safety and efficacy of medication, has not approved bioidentical hormones, and many health insurance companies do not cover them. In contrast, medications that Western doctors prescribe have been properly tested in reliable medical studies, proving their safety and efficacy as per the FDA. Compounded bioidenticals have also not been tested in clinical trials in the same manner as hormone replacement therapy. Then there's the question of what is "natural?" Are bioidenticals more "natural?" They're made from plant products such as soy and yams, but they still need chemical processing to become active in the body. In truth, many estrogen pills, patches, gels, creams and sprays are also bioidentical, so just because hormones are termed bioidentical, it doesn't mean that they are more natural.

My point is that if you do choose to use bioidentical hormones, it's important to understand that they are not proven to be any safer than hormone replacement therapy.

In Gretchen's case, she was given too much estrogen and, as a result, developed pre-cancer cells of the uterus. As for the monitoring of her estrogen, salivary testing has not been shown to be a reliable way of testing estrogen levels in the body. The good news is that pre-cancer cells are a medically treatable condition, but one that could have been prevented if Gretchen had been prescribed a safer, lower dose of HRT.

The Emotional Side of Mature V

In addition to the hot flashes, irregular periods, and insomnia linked to menopause, there are mental changes proven to be equally frustrating and downright depressing. The low estrogen levels that cause menopausal symptoms can also cause drops in serotonin and dopamine levels, leading to depression and other cognitive changes, including memory loss, poor concentration, and short attention span. Going through the process myself, I can truthfully say that those cognitive changes, especially memory loss, are the most disruptive and frustrating of menopause.

A woman's natural estrogen supply is protection against depression, a common menopausal symptom. The severity of depression varies, depending on a number of factors and life circumstances. A key hormonal milestone such as menopause (as well as pregnancy or puberty) influences a woman's level of depression, anxiety, or mood changes. Menopause can worsen a woman's existing tendency towards depression or bring upon depression for the first time, for which I would recommend hormone replacement therapy as a first line of defense *before* prescribing antidepressants. However, as far as the feelings of forgetfulness and lack of focus are concerned, there may well be other factors in play.

ADHD and ADD medications can be helpful with menopausal symptoms related to focus, organization, time management, and forgetfulness, also known as "foggy brain." Even if you haven't been officially diagnosed with ADHD in the past, menopause can throw you into an ADHD-like state. I have a handful of patients who take ADHD medications to control their cognitive changes so they can feel like life hasn't taken a turn for the worse, but it's important that potential ADD sufferers be diagnosed by the right healthcare provider, which, traditionally, is *not* a gynecologist. That said, the first conversation you have may well be with your gynecologist, who may then be able to recommend a next step.

Take control of the direction in which your mature vagina is headed. Don't back down from or be afraid of the natural changes life has in store for us. For most of us at this juncture, life is happening full throttle. The stresses of relationships, children, aging parents, and work accumulate with age. I hear the menopausal battle cries of "I'm going F**KING crazy!" in my examining room and on the phone with my closest friends. Sixty percent of this group of women are going through a divorce or have kids going off to college (or kids coming home after finding out that college is not for them), or have job worries. The advice I share with all the women in my life is to first and foremost be honest with yourself and listen to what your body is saying. Increase the quality of your own life. If you are suffering from menopausal symptoms there are safe treatments available for you. Your healthcare provider should be educating you on options, and if they aren't, it's up to you to find another provider. In order to be the best version of yourself to deal with your own life, you need to be in control of your mental and physical state. You must be your own best health advocate, regardless of age... and hormonal status.

I want to hear you and your Mature V roar back at menopause!

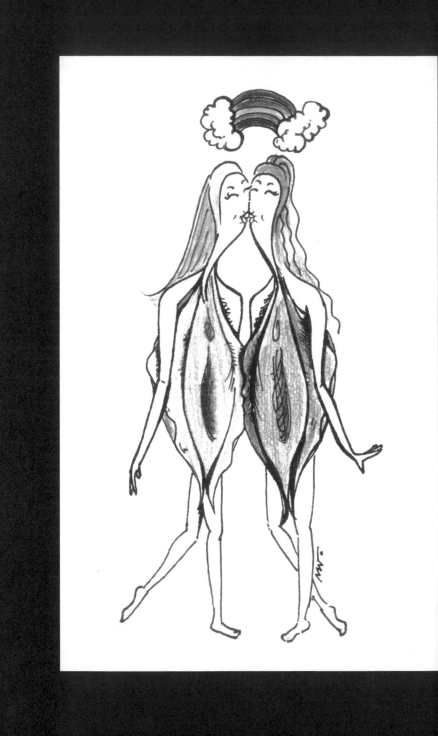

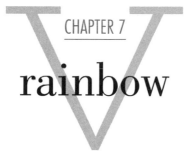

CHAPTER 7

rainbow

❝As a little girl with two older brothers and a disconnected mother, I had no concept of what constituted being a girl. I just knew I wasn't a boy, which meant I didn't have a handy penis and couldn't pee standing up, I wasn't as strong or as fast or as vocal as the boys, and I understood my opinion didn't matter as much as theirs.

I remember the first time I really saw my vagina… I must have been about five, on my back, on the floor, my feet planted high up against the closet mirror; I was horrified. It was the most hideous thing I'd ever seen. Nothing neatly packaged and interactive like what boys got to play with…I just had flaps, folds, and a hole!

I didn't know if God was real (although I'd heard his name bandied about in my family) but I was sure he had made a terrible mistake. I didn't know if anyone else had noticed but there was no doubt that what *I* had was not meant to happen!

She-ology

There was no one to compare it to, no one to complain to. It's sad to think back at how the years of harboring threads of those childish feelings allowed them to meld, unchallenged by any counter opinion, into a subtle sense of feeling sexually unattractive, undesirable, and inadequate. I always understood that the power was in the penis. I never really wanted a penis but I depended on the power attached to it.

As an aloof, lonely young woman, I had a desperate need to be loved, to prove myself sexually, therefore worthy. Many familial factors contributed to this, of course, but the underpinning of my alliances was initially fueled more by desperation than attraction. I used sex as a tool to manipulate and control meaningless male encounters so I'd feel validated. The fact that I wasn't particularly attracted during these hook-ups didn't weigh on me; that was never the goal.

I married at nineteen, which was like being adrift in an unwelcome sea and coming upon a prickly log, which I hoped could keep me afloat. I didn't wait for a different kind of log; I just grabbed on and kept my chin up. Over the years, several such logs bobbed my way. Lucky me.

Cut to thirty years, three husbands, and five children later, I meet a woman who turns my head around. She is twenty-five years my junior…young enough for me to realize it could never go much beyond the OH-MY-GOD-I'M-A-LESBIAN moment…and the relationship dies a sad little death. But I do NOT. The penny has dropped; the ship has sailed; the coop is flown; a 55-year-old baby dyke is born!

One upside of this is that I never dealt with the shame, confusion, pain and fear so many young people suffered in their struggles with sexual identity. I never had to come out to my parents. The downside of this is I felt the shame and confusion of being the least self-examined person on the earth to not have at least *questioned* my sexuality before I was halfway through my sixth decade.

Rainbow V

Thankfully, I worked with my therapist, addressing the thinking behind my relationships with men as I started dating women. I'd developed lots of unattractive defensive behaviors I didn't want to carry into new liaisons; I Roto-Rootered my brain.

My formal coming out (which happened the way it does for so many of us, *The Today Show* with a spread in *People* magazine) didn't send my career up in flames as I feared. I experienced a warm welcome from the gay community and a few lifted brows of surprise from the straight. Other than those sad trolls that just have to say something miserable, it wasn't the difficult time I'd anticipated. My family and friends had known for years and that helped.

I felt unburdened and accepted and if I wasn't accepted, *I didn't care.* My girl Nancy and I have been together more than ten years and married two-and-a-half. To be a wife with a wife is a wonderful thing; we revel that we are pioneers among other like pioneers. "

—Meredith Baxter Actress & Producer

"When I was in medical school I thought I was destined to be a pediatrician. That was before I spent twelve weeks on the obstetrics and gynecology rotation at Metropolitan Hospital in Harlem, New York. In those three months I not only assisted in eight major surgeries, I delivered ten babies by myself. The babies are what did it. I knew afterwards that my calling was to bring children into this world and to help women find strength through the health and awareness of their own reproductive organs—including, of course, their vaginas.

If you missed it in my introduction to this book, I am a lesbian OB-GYN. Maybe it's because of my sexual orientation—or maybe it's the unavoidable genetics of the nurturing Jewish mother—but I have always been ultra-sensitive to my patients' feelings and needs. First and foremost, I try to make my patients comfortable in their exams and comfortable in discussing any issue with me, medical or otherwise. I'm blessed with new patients who somehow find their way to my office, and patients who have been coming to me since I started private practice some twenty-five years ago. During any given routine appointment, the conversation may cover everything from vaginas, to work, to aging parents, to whatever life stresses have evolved since a previous visit. Invariably, a patient will ask me about my family, and—in the case of relatively new patients—what my "husband" does. At that point I have to make a quick judgment call. Do I say, "Well, my wife is a high school principal in Watts," or do I change the subject?

Now, don't get me wrong. I am a loud, proud, and "out" lesbian, but it is my job to make a new patient feel safe and comfortable, and my quick judgment has everything to do with just that. You may say, "But you're a doctor! What difference does it make?" And, of course, I would argue that it makes no difference, but if a male gynecologist is about to examine a patient, a female nurse is required to be in the room with him to ensure that there isn't any inappropriate touching. Here's the thing: Many years ago I had a new patient, Bonnie. When she asked about my spouse, I told her what her name was. Bonnie stuttered a bit, then said, "But you don't look like a lesbian. And you have three boys! Huh. My friend who recommended you didn't mention that you were lesbian." Well, that was Bonnie's last visit with me.

I live a life as true to myself as possible, but as a doctor who examines naked women, it is vital to establish a bond of trust and comfort with my patients. Yes, I'm afraid there is a double standard, obviously, because most of the male gynecologists I know are straight. But being an openly lesbian gynecologist is, in the scheme of things, relatively new. There are still an awful lot of myths amongst heterosexuals that make me more than a little wary about exposing my personal behavior.

I promise you, I still hear arguments such as "If you're a lesbian, it's because you've never had a meaningful relationship with a man." Or "I've heard that lesbians can't help but be attracted to other women, even if they are in long-term relationships." So the truth is that I probably go a bit overboard in making my patients feel as comfortable as possible when I'm in the situation of having to come in for a close-up between their legs. If I could, I would offer my patients tea and cookies while they're in the stirrups, just to be a good host!

Which is to say that my first priority is giving my patients not only the best care possible, but also the respect and compassion that women need and deserve. I reach out to my LGBT community because they are the minority, the underdogs in receiving medical care and gainful employment. I am advocate, friend and physician to this community I call family. If I'm lucky I can help make their lives just a little easier. 99

—**Dr. Sherry** OB-GYN, Women's Health Expert, Author

Girls Like Girls

It may or may not surprise you to know that one in ten girls is sexually attracted to other girls. As adolescents, personal sexuality is completely confusing since our only understanding of sex comes from what we see and hear in movies, on TV, from social media, or older siblings or friends. As a high school athlete I was aware of my own attraction to my coaches and teammates. What did that mean, I wondered? Watching Mariel Hemingway as an athlete who falls in love with her female teammate in the 1982 movie *Personal Best* (radical, at the time!) I was alternately "grossed out" and secretly fascinated. Melissa Etheridge came out in the 80s, and I loved her music, but there were very few lesbians in the mainstream media, especially lesbians who weren't decidedly (and comically) butch. Like many teens seeking truth in love and sexuality, I was confused. I dated men, and I even married one, and then I had three sons in quick succession (for which I will be forever grateful). But now, after eight years of marriage to my wife Peggy, I can honestly say I never had the emotional, physical, and sexual connection with any other person in my life as I do with her. It's my wish that every woman, gay or straight, find unconditional love in a partner at some juncture in her life. Ladies, you deserve to be loved for who you are; there is no greater gift!

It's *Your* Health Care

The National Survey of Family Growth suggests that 1.1 percent of women identify themselves as lesbian, and 3.5 percent of women identify as bisexual. Historically, lesbian and bisexual women have felt afraid and apprehensive about getting health care because of confidentiality and disclosure, discriminatory attitudes and treatment, uncertainty about their healthcare needs and risks, and because of limited access to health care and health insurance. Know your rights. The bottom line is that all healthcare providers must provide the same complete medical care to lesbian, bisexual, transgender, and heterosexual women.

Healthcare providers are often uncomfortable asking questions directly related to sexual orientation, but these specific questions are important and necessary in providing proper preventive care and treatment. When you're having your medical and sexual history taken by your healthcare provider, they may overlook your sexual orientation. A "yes" to the question of "Are you sexually active?" needs to be followed up with "Are you sexually active with a male or female?" A lesbian may not offer the information unless she is asked directly, and if there's no exchange of this vital information, there is no real communication between patient and healthcare provider. I believe the medical community needs to take the lead and learn the appropriate and sensitive way of asking the potentially uncomfortable medical questions necessary to bridge the gap in a doctor-patient relationship, especially concerning lesbian and bisexual patients.

Studies in the past have found that lesbians and bisexual women have higher health risks than heterosexual women and a greater incidence of the following:

* Obesity
* Tobacco use
* Alcohol and drug use
* Type 2 Adult Onset Diabetes
* Lung cancer
* Cardiac disease and heart attacks

Whatever the factors in these health concerns (perhaps depression caused by alienation or discrimination?), it is important for lesbians to be aware of their increased health risks and even more important for them to disclose their sexual orientation to their healthcare provider so that they may provide the appropriate medical screenings.

It's essential that a lesbian or bisexual woman find a healthcare provider with whom she feels completely comfortable. And that comfort needs to extend to a welcoming and receptive office staff as well.

Reproductive Rights

On June 26, 2015, the U.S. Supreme Court ruled that gay marriage is a right protected by the United States Constitution in all fifty states. A long time coming, indeed. Public opinion finds a sixty percent approval of gay marriage compared to twenty-seven percent twenty years ago. Although this seems like an equitable gain, I'd say we're still short about forty percent!

Since same-sex marriage is now legal, employment rights and benefits now, thankfully, include lesbians, gay couples, and domestic partnership. That said, some health providers will not provide fertility services to women who identify themselves as lesbian. These providers seem to think that the families in the LGBT community must be guided by different rules and guidelines than heterosexual couples. But sexual orientation should never be a barrier to receiving fertility treatments. The American College of Obstetricians and Gynecologists backs me up on this one. The College "endorses equitable treatment for lesbians and their families, not only for direct healthcare needs, but also for indirect healthcare issues; this should include the same legal protections afforded married couples."

66 Having children wasn't something that Kelly or I had thought much about until we met, fell in love, and started building a life together. We were both very driven and ambitious career women, but once we settled down and bought a house—decorated it together and filled it with pets—we had the conversation about whether or not to have children. It was the success of our relationship that inspired us to start our family and made us feel confident that we could provide

a loving home as two same-sex parents. Since I'm the "older one" (by a mere five years) Kelly and I decided that I would "go first"—that is, be the first of us to become pregnant since we wanted to have two children. After carefully considering our options we agreed to use the same unknown donor for both children.

Unfortunately, the fertility clinics and their doctors we hired to handle our inseminations were unsupportive emotionally. It felt like a factory. We couldn't wait until that part of the process was over. Fortunately, when we got pregnant, we found ourselves in the experienced and compassionate hands of Dr. Sherry Ross and her nurse Danielle. They took such good care of us and made both our pregnancy experiences a pleasure.

In August of 2001 our first daughter was born. Four years later Kelly gave birth to our second daughter, and I ended up quitting my job in order for one of us to be one hundred percent available to our kids. I speak for both Kelly and I when I say that raising our two amazing girls has been the best (and hardest) thing either of us has ever done. Parenting has not only brought us closer to each other, it has helped us discover one of our greatest joys in life...being soccer moms! Both our families are supportive of our children and us, and we're happy to report that our kids have grandparents as proud and boastful of them as the next kids' grandmas and grandpas.

We have always been honest with our daughters about how they were conceived, and we gladly answer any questions they have. They, in turn, are proud of having two moms—when they were young we heard from several preschool parents that their kids came home asking why *they* couldn't also have two moms! Since we live in Los Angeles, several of our daughters' peers have either two moms or two dads, but I think it's also a case of the world changing (for the better) in regards to acceptance of same-sex parents.

We were among the first of our lesbian friends to have children. It was before same-sex marriage was legal, so we had to first become domestic partners and then hire a lawyer and go to court to adopt the daughter we didn't give birth to—a tedious time and money-consuming process. Millennial lesbian couples have it so much easier!

We cannot imagine our life without our daughters, and we are proud of the compassionate young women they are becoming. Also, we are happy to rely on the continued guidance of Dr. Sherry Ross— we can only hope she'll still be in practice when *they're* ready to have children! **99**

—**Kelly & Linda Novak** Mothers to Ava and Zoe

Family Planning

Same-sex couples are getting married, planning families, and trying to live their American Dream, but the truth is that for the LGBT community, the dream is more complicated than for most Americans. Google "lesbians and conception" and the information that pops up on your home page is pretty disappointing. The hundreds of lesbian couples who have been in my care over the past twenty-four years can attest to that dearth of information. Fortunately, I've been able to fill in some fairly large gaps, the biggest of which is often around the topic of emotional readiness.

Just because you *can* conceive, doesn't necessarily mean that you should, or that you are ready. You and your partner need to do the homework and research on what it takes to plan for a family, including the financial commitment of pregnancy and raising a child (or two). This process alone can lead to a lot of stress (sometimes, depression) for one or both of you. Lengthy conversations regarding the process, from start to finish, are vital. These conversations must cover who will carry the pregnancy, whose egg will be used and *where the sperm is coming from*—don't forget, that's half the recipe. Will the sperm be from a known or direct donor, or from an anonymous donor? I recommend making a long list of questions to address in this stressful process.

The stress is no joke. Studies have shown that straight couples are three times more likely to divorce or becomes separated after failed fertility treatments—obviously it's too soon for accurate statistics on LGBT couples—and that the most challenging time for couples is the transition to parenthood. If a couple had marital problems before the challenges of the fertility process, then they would likely continue to struggle with the same issues throughout the fertility process and beyond. Some lesbian couples have found it immensely helpful to see a therapist prior to beginning the fertility journey.

Once you've embarked on the journey, it's imperative to find an OB-GYN. I realize that here in Los Angeles I have easy, open access to a very large gay community, which, in turn, has made *me* accessible to the community. As a lesbian doctor, I feel a great responsibility to reach out to what has historically been a largely underserved, undereducated, and underrepresented group of people. In whatever city you may reside, find an OB-GYN who is comfortable in dealing with lesbians, and who may foster a positive and supportive environment from beginning to end. I would suggest contacting your city's LGBT community or health center to find out whom they might recommend. Talk to friends who have been through the process. Get their recommendations. For your experience to be a positive one, not only do your expectations need to be realistic, the whole shebang must be cost effective.

Your Gynecologic Care

I knew that Michelle, a 45-year old professor at USC's Women's Studies Department with an infectious smile and a confident stride, was "family" as soon as she sat down in my office for her first visit. Tall, lean, in a blue, tailored suit matching piercing blue eyes, she had been referred to me by a group of lesbian women patients from West Hollywood. Admittedly, she'd not been to a gynecologist in five years. Newly single after a seven-year relationship, not only had she never had a pelvic exam, but she'd never had a mammogram! Her reason: "I don't have any problems with my periods and no family history of cancer, so I didn't think I needed to come in unless I was having problems.... I see an Eastern medicine doctor every few months for back pain from having played professional beach volleyball, but the pain has gotten progressively worse." I guess I wasn't very good at keeping my astonishment at bay because she continued, "Honestly, it was my understanding that I didn't need to worry about Pap smears and sexually transmitted infections since I'm a lesbian." This coming from a woman with a PhD.

Along with lesbian patients, many gynecologists are not clear as to when Pap smear screenings ought to begin and how often they need be done. The thinking remains: Since lesbians aren't having sex with men, they don't need Pap smears, right? Wrong. This is a complete misconception. Lesbians do need to have routine Pap smears, along with regular gynecological visits.

Rainbow V

Many lesbians have been sexually active with men in their pasts. One study involving 6,000 lesbians found that seventy-seven percent have had sex with men and that seventy percent reported a lifetime history of vaginal intercourse. Aside from those statistics, female-to-female sexual activity still puts lesbians at risk for STIs that include bacterial vaginosis, candidiasis, herpes, and HPV—news flash: lesbians get HPV, too!—all of which increase the risk for abnormal Pap smears. Regardless of sexual orientation, the practice of safe sex in reducing the risk of transmitting or acquiring STIs should be encouraged.

Now that you know that STIs are equal opportunity infections, I can't stress the fact enough that HPV is the most common STI in women and men. Unfortunately, studies show that lesbians have been much less likely to be educated on HPV and the importance of vaccinations against this infection. Female-to-female transmission through sexual activity is one way this highly contagious virus is passed to women, which increases the risk of cervical cancer. Lesbian, bisexual, and transgender women and men should receive the HPV vaccine, ideally between the ages of eleven and twenty-six.

Also more prevalent among lesbians than heterosexual women: Nullgravity (no history of pregnancy), obesity, tobacco use, and less use of oral contraception. Any of these factors alone or combined are associated with an increased risk of breast and ovarian cancer.

As I told Michelle, lesbians and bisexual women need to see a healthcare provider or gynecologist with the same frequency as heterosexual women. Whether you are gay or straight, the Pap smear, breast and pelvic examinations, and mammograms are done at the same regular intervals.

Screenings for osteoporosis, colorectal cancer, and mental health (including intimate partner violence) are also an important part of regular physicals.

Fun But Safe

Despite her petite 5'3" frame, Dre (short for Andrea) walks through my practice like she's six feet tall. I don't think I've ever seen Dre out of her "uniform" of Levi's 501's, wife-beater tee and baseball cap (worn sideways), and I've never caught her in a down mood. She'd recently returned from the Dinah Shore Golf Tournament in Palm Springs and was in my office regaling me with the details of her non-stop party weekend with her girlfriend of three months. Fun to hear, but, whoa, did I feel old. It sounded like she'd never slept, on top of having "had the best sex of [her] life." It was the first time she and her partner hadn't used a dental dam, the first time they'd "fisted" each other, and, unfortunately, the first time Dre had ended up with some sort of funky vaginal discharge. Thank goodness she was so candid about her sexual adventures, if only because it made it easier for me to diagnose the source of her problem. It seemed that not only did Dre have small tears at the entrance of her vagina, she'd also picked up a nasty bacterial infection. I was able to prescribe the proper course of treatment and send her on her way to another weekend of sexual fireworks. **VVL**

Regardless of your sexual orientation, safe sex practices should be discussed and encouraged in order to reduce the risk of giving or receiving STIs and HIV. For lesbian and bisexual women, safe sex includes condoms for sex toys, gloves for "fisting" (putting a fist into the vagina or anus), dental dams for oral sex, and the proper cleaning of sex toys and dildos *between* partners.

Gay, straight, bisexual or transgender—the same level of respect, patience, openness and understanding should be given to all by *every* member of the medical community.

Despite a drastically improved rate of acceptance for the LGBT community in the last few years, many lesbians still have a difficult time being "out" in the world. Fortunately, there are many courageous LGBT public figures that continue to speak out for their peers.

Influential and Gay

And then came Ellen! Dietram Scheufele, a communications professor at the University of Wisconsin noted, "Ellen DeGeneres is...almost a litmus test of where we have been as a society. When she first came out and really put the issue of same-sex partnerships on people's agendas—and I mean people who really wouldn't have thought about it—I think the country was still in a very different state."

Closeted to the world for the majority of her life, Ellen "came out" in 1997 on primetime TV on her titular sitcom. *Time Magazine* promptly put her on their cover even while sponsors for the show pulled their advertising. But mainstream America mostly followed with overwhelming love and support—evidently, as *The Ellen Degeneres Show* is now in its fourteenth season.

I have to acknowledge another champion of culture change, Ilene Chaiken, who created *The L Word*, which was the groundbreaking lesbian drama that forced everyone to see the LGBTQ community through a more positive and mainstream lens.

She-ology

Other women in Hollywood who have been loudly proud and truthful about their sexual identity include Melissa Etheridge, Meredith Baxter, Leisha Hailey, Lily Tomlin, Cynthia Nixon, Wanda Sykes, Suze Orman, Guinevere Turner, Rachel Maddow, Rosie O'Donnell, Clementine Ford, Ruby Rose, Alexandra Hedison, Elizabeth Keener, Jodie Foster, and Ellen Page.

"My parents always nurtured my artistic side. They tried to instill in me the belief that individuality was important, that it was brave to go against the norm, and that by standing out, I could become a leader. So I can only wonder when and where self-hatred entered into my life. When did I turn on the one thing I could depend upon—myself?

I grew up in a small town—which served primarily as an Air Force Base—and took on the role of *tomboy* very early on. Although I had *odd feelings* regarding other girls, I instinctively knew to keep those feelings to myself. Year after year it became more apparent that conforming to the norm was easier than challenging it. So I went on dates, I had boyfriends, and I smiled my way through my seventeen years of *normalcy*. I turned to the television to find a role model. I searched for a mentor among my teachers, someone I could talk to about my true feelings and who would give me permission to be myself. I looked to my friends and their parents for some subtle message of: *It's okay, you can tell me. It's safe.*

But no one provided that message. So I did what any self-deprecating teenager does: I swallowed all of my feelings. It seemed better to hide my little gay self away and deal with her another time. I continued to be a normal, happy teenager—one who was dying inside. *I must be a freak*, I thought. My primary job became that of handling my secret, keeping it hidden. But, I imagined, one day... one day I would feel free.

Rainbow V

When I moved to New York City, I waited for that freedom to set in. But it didn't. I waited for the world to say, "We love you! We love who you are and we love that you're different!" But that didn't happen. And then it hit me; my job was not to keep my secret, but to share it. How could I expect the world to embrace me with open arms if I didn't fully love myself first? How could I expect someone else, someone other than me, to magically erase my own shame and fear?

I realized I couldn't rely on anyone else to do my work *for* me. I needed courage in the belief that my differences were extraordinarily beautiful and powerful, and that by being proud of who I was I would, in some small way, help to change the world. I knew in my heart that true transformation came about by example. I knew that I had to set a standard for the world I wanted to live in. Leaders bring other leaders into existence. I sought to find my community so that together we could forge a new path. By loving our gay selves, we demand the respect we deserve, and in that love, hate cannot penetrate.

As I have watched the world change before my eyes, I've become proud and grateful to be gay. The sisterhood moves dauntlessly forward with leaders in many aspects, one of whom, Dr. Sherry Ross, happened to write this book. Far and wide, here and throughout the world, we walk forward together. 🙶

—**Leisha Hailey** Actress & Musician

For many LGBTQ people, their sexual orientation was known to them early on; sometimes as far back as they can remember. For others it was a less obvious and more gradual understanding. Whether your own revelation came before or after puberty, it is known that a person's sexual orientation is a result of biologic, hereditary, and environmental influences. Regardless of your age, if you are struggling to understand your own sexual identity it's important to understand that you are completely normal in your confusion. The care of your body and mental and sexual health all carry equal weight. Being in touch with your feelings and asking the hard questions must be a priority. Reach out to friends, and then find a reliable and trusted medical professional.

I remember sitting down with my best friends and telling them I was not only divorcing my husband—for issues that actually had nothing to do with my sexuality—I was going to follow my heart and date women. Not surprisingly, my BFFs barely blinked at my revelations (a reminder of how well they knew me). In my utter relief and gratitude of their support we had one of the most fun and memorable evenings of our friendships—although I have to admit that the bottomless margaritas didn't hurt. The truth is your best friends will love you unconditionally and may be your greatest source of encouragement.

Lesbian, bisexual, transgender, and heterosexual vaginas all have the same gynecological health and medical needs. Demand respect from your healthcare providers, and, more to the point, give your body, your soul and your vagina the respect they deserve. Claim the person you are and love them for life.

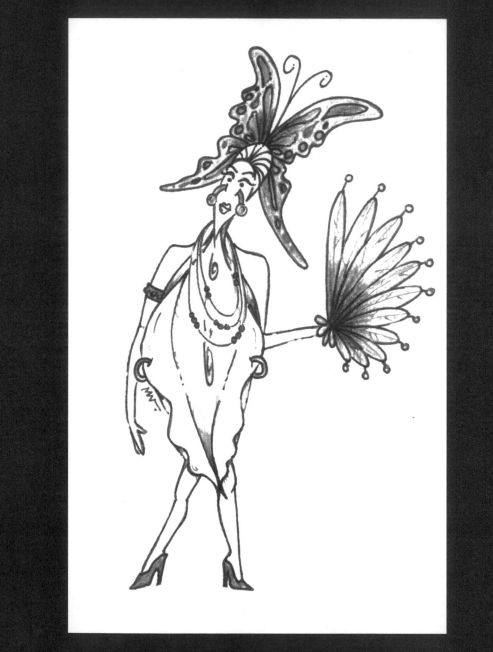

CHAPTER 8

glamorous

> I've been in the beauty industry as a professional makeup artist longer than I care to mention. Having worked on many different faces, all different shapes, tones and sizes, *I believe that beauty ultimately comes from within. A woman's confidence and strength manifests in the beauty of one's own personal style.*

By personal style, I mean the way in which you express yourself feels harmonious with your true self and staying true to your own style, no matter what it may be.

As far as your V is concerned, again, it's your personal preference in how far you want to go. You may be the only person who sees your V, but if that's where you want to express your original style then do it. Go for a glamorous V if that's what you want. Play around with the shape and color. There are many choices from wide to a natural outline or a thinner more manicured V, all the way to bare skin. It really depends on what makes you feel sexy and comfortable in your body.

She·ology

No matter your "look," I would suggest a few simple things in order to *maintain* that beautiful, unique style of yours—call it advice from a beauty pro if you want. Here goes: More water. Less booze. No smokes. Regular facials. Sun block—always. No Botox before thirty! And don't forget: Self-expression can happen anywhere on your body, as evident in the Glamorous V.

[From Dr. Sherry: *Jillian won't mention this, but she's flown all over the world to do make up on the likes of Jennifer Lawrence and Kristen Stewart (among others). Jillian evidently loves her work, because every time she comes for her gynecologic exam, she pulls a few goodies out of her magic makeup bag and reapplies my eyeliner, puts blush on my cheeks, colors in my brows, and assesses my colorist's latest work on my hair! It's a nice bonus, being attended to, especially by one of the most sought-after makeup artists in Hollywood!*] 🙶

—Jillian Dempsey Professional Makeup Artist

At fifty-one, Alison was four years out of her long-time marriage to her high school boyfriend. She was the kind of mom I wished I could have been—generous with her time, a volunteer in every school event and parent association, baker of home-made double chocolate chip cookies, and Girl Scout Leader (twelve years running!). Along with all that, Alison managed to keep a fitness-trainer physique. You'd want to be her or hate her, but she was so genuinely lovely that you couldn't help but want her as a friend, or, at least, on your kids' fundraising committee. During her latest annual visit, she told me, excitedly, "I've just started dating again! Crazy, but I haven't done anything to my pubic hair in years, except maybe for some summer bathing suit trims. Seriously, I want my vagina to look 2016 and not so 1986! What do I do? I mean, how can I glam it up or 'vajazzle the punai,' as my daughter puts it?"

These days there are many fashionable choices for your vagina and pubic hair. Some women think a little grooming goes a long way, others go all out in hair removal, tattooing, or piercing, and still others will tell you that a clean vagina is good enough. It's personal opinion at best. Whether you're stuck in 70s "full bush" fashion and considering a modern alternative, or you're hoping to spice up your sex life with something more vagina edgy or glamorous, here's a look into today's vag fashions and trends.

What Is the Purpose of Pubic Hair?

No one really knows the official purpose of pubic hair, but there are some *theories.*

Pubic hair: (1) prevents dirt from entering the vagina, (2) keeps the genitals warm, (3) acts as a cushion during sex, spinning, soul cycling, and other forms of exercise, (4) creates sex pheromones, which are erotic smells that excite a partner, (5) depending upon the culture, is solely of decorative value.

If you have a theory of your own, I'd be happy to hear it!

Birth of the Mod-Glam Vagina

Sharon Stone (in *Basic Instinct*): "It's nice."

Yes, indeed, the sexual innuendo was unmistakable when, in 1992, Ms. Stone uncrossed her legs in the infamous interrogation scene revealing her coiffed vagina while uttering those two little words. It was mainstream movie history and it viscerally impacted its audience, men and women alike. Many agreed it *was* nice, if not jarring, but it certainly ushered in glamorous Vs for a conventional audience.

It used to be that porn stars and swimsuit models were the only ones coifing their vaginas, but now, in 2017, American women consider grooming their vagina—in the case of trimming, waxing or laser removal of pubic hair—as part of their regular beauty regimen, along with manis and pedis, brow/lip/leg waxing, and eyelash tinting.

It seems there are a variety of reasons why **women like to groom their pubic hair**. Ask a roomful of us and this is what you may hear:

* Less hair means less bush!
* I think a waxed vagina looks more clean and tidy—and I can show off my "lady luscious labia."
* My boyfriend likes it gone. My husband likes it trimmed. (And, no, I don't know if this was spoken by the same women.)
* It's sexier!
* It looks and feels better!
* It's better for oral sex.
* It's better if you want to wear a bathing suit without a towel wrapped around your waist all day.
* Definitely better for G-strings and edible underwear.
* I feel more sensual when my vagina's waxed, and it makes my orgasms more intense.
* Less hair means fewer vaginal odors and skin irritations (spoken like a true pragmatist).

In a recent survey 5,000 men were asked, "What do you find attractive when it comes to women's pubic hair?"

Glamorous V

Forty-one percent preferred the "completely bare look," noting that, "Brazilian is king!" (More on *the Brazilian* in a bit.) Thirty-eight percent preferring a trimmed and well-groomed pubic area, citing that a grown woman ought to have "something down there." Fifteen percent had no preference whatsoever; generously acknowledging "a woman should do whatever makes her feel comfortable and sexy." Five percent preferred an "all natural" bush, and one percent said "other" (whatever that might mean).

Although eighty-five percent of the men surveyed did, indeed, have a preference when it came to a woman's pubic hair, only nine percent claimed they would end a date or that they would forego sex based on a woman's care of her pubic hair. Even as of this writing, the style tending towards a bit more bush may be trending.

It seems that the American Apparel store in New York City prefers a little pubic hair, as is demonstrated in their new storefront mannequins. The clothing giant has always loved playing with the definition of what is feminine and sexy. With the "bush additions" to their window displays, they appear to be dispelling the look as unnatural and unhygienic. Are the 70s back, or have they never gone? Apparently, American Apparel is onto something since Lady Gaga asked to have one of the mannequins bearing a full bush join her on her music tour. All of this isn't to suggest that men are left out of the grooming trends.

It may surprise you, but eighty-eight percent of men do some form of manscaping (defined as the aesthetic grooming of a man's bodily hair). Out of this percentage, nearly half felt the pressure to do some pubic grooming because their partner did so. But what really impressed me about this study was that two-thirds of the men surveyed found that a woman who didn't fuss about grooming and who was comfortable in her own skin to be sexier than a woman who put excessive time and money into trying to maintain someone else's idea of perfection. Interesting. Three cheers for these particular men!

As for my own first waxing experience: I remember approaching it armed with a headful of nightmarish stories about waxes gone horribly bad. I was preparing for my second marriage and I wanted to surprise my wife by getting *it all* removed for our honeymoon in Bora Bora. Hard to believe, after seeing hundreds of wax jobs in my practice, that I'd never done anything more creative than the mundane bathing suit wax, which constituted a neat, conservative suit-line trim. But I had a patient who managed Queen Bee Waxing, the best waxing salon in nearby Culver City, and she assured me that it wouldn't be bad, that it would, in fact, "be fun!" I held my judgment and followed all her pre-waxing tips, including the application of a numbing cream one hour before my appointment. Okay, I have to say now that it wasn't all bad, but I wouldn't describe it as "fun" either. Awkward might be the best way to describe how I felt. Needless to say, I didn't anticipate the acrobatic positions I'd have to assume so that waxer/owner extraordinaire Jodie could reach *all* the hair. When she told me to get on all fours I had to squelch the urge to crawl on hands and knees out the door. Fortunately, that stance heralded the grand finale.

To be honest, a Pap smear is a whole lot more *fun* than a full Brazilian—but that's just me.

And while we're on the subject...

Waxing

You know the term (and have probably suffered or enjoyed at least a session or two). It refers to a form of grooming in which pubic hair is *temporarily* removed from its root. Since the lifecycle of hair is approximately four to six weeks, it takes that same amount of time for the hair to return. This common form of grooming is relatively quick and painless (unless you're me). Warm wax is applied to the pubic hair that is to be removed using a small strip of cloth. Once the wax hardens, the cloth is yanked off along with the unwanted hair. Voila! There can be redness and pain associated with this particular beautifying procedure, but take hope as there are numbing creams that can be applied to the vagina and pubic hair area to make the procedure less uncomfortable.

Like any good hairstyle, there are a number of variations to *the wax*. First off, if you're immune to waxing styles, be assured that there's always The Natural Bush. No hair is removed (or harmed) in the making of this *au natural* style. No trimming, no muss, no fuss. The big and bushy trend is always on its way in (or out). Short of letting it all hang out is to simply **trim** pubic hair, which involves only shortening the hair. As far as **waxing styles**, there are a few: **VVL**

* **Triangle** or **bikini line waxing**: this removes pubic hair, leaving the remaining hair in the shape of a neat triangle so that when you wear a swimsuit there is nothing visible. Another name for this type of wax job is The Bermuda Triangle. A smaller such triangle is a Martini (no olive).
* **American waxing**, referred to as a **basic bikini wax**, is the removal of any pubic hair that might be seen

when wearing a swimsuit. This may include removal of hair on the upper thighs.

* **French waxing** is a type of pubic hair removal that leaves a vertical strip. It's also known as the **Landing** or **Playboy strip** or a **partial Brazilian** wax. It leaves a strip of hair just above the vulva about two inches long and an inch and a half wide. Anal hair as well as pubic hair is removed in this type of wax job. A fuller version of the narrow strip is a **Mohawk**.

* The **full-bush Brazilian** is the removal of all pubic and anal hair—ouch. Pardon me—although sometimes a very thin strip of hair is left on the pubic area. Bikini waxer extraordinaire Jola Brozdynski describes the full-bush Brazilian as the wax job "for Hippies with porn-y sex lives." Those worshippers of the hairless look claim that sex is better on every level, especially with oral sex. Obviously, a mouthful of hair is not an issue after a Brazilian. If you were to listen to Eva Longoria's advice, you must try a Brazilian at least once in your life. Apparently, the sex you'll have in the wake of such a wax will keep you coming back again and again.

Other creative styles include The Romantic, also known as The Heart or Heart Attack, which leaves the pubic hair in the shape of a heart—a popular Valentine's Day pattern. The French may refer to their pubic wax as an **Underground Ticket** or **Ticket de Metro**.

Japanese Fan, Square Style, Short and Sweet, Very Vivacious, Sphinx Style, The Directive, The Gambler, The Bare-Cheeked Butler, The Excuse, The Patriot, Freestyle and

Hollywood are other names I've heard mentioned over the years and in my research. Go ahead, pick a name, whatever it may be, there's a long line of female (and male) waxing fans. So while we're at it...

The Benefits of Waxing

There are definitely fewer incidences of ingrown hairs in waxing, as compared with shaving the sensitive pubic area. Hair regrowth after waxing also tends to be softer. (Globally, Bikini waxing has also resulted in a decrease in pubic lice!) If you are bold enough, you may do a bikini wax in the privacy of your own home. With experience, you'll become a little more skilled with each rip—er, I mean, removal. Waxing hair in the pubic area may also prove a kinder and gentler effect on the skin of the vagina as you can wait four to six weeks in between waxing sessions, thereby causing less skin aggravation.

Disadvantages?

I love witnessing my bright young patients grow up and have children—as was the case with Olivia. Now thirty-two, she's been my patient since she was eighteen. Creative and impulsive, she was equally so with her vagina. Olivia could have been poster girl for "patterns in pubic hair waxing." She was especially proud of the time she dyed her pubic hair bright red in honor of Valentine's Day. At her six-week postpartum visit, after delivery of her second daughter, Olivia insisted that she needed to be "vagina ready" to resume sex with her husband, Jeff— after all, Jeff was quick to remind her that it had been seven weeks and four days of abstinence—so she made an appointment with a "wax technician" at the newly opened and as yet untried Pink Cheeks salon. After the date, Olivia came to see me with a three-inch laceration along the fold of her labia which had been bleeding on and off since her waxing a few days before. Yes, the point is that sometimes waxing has its complications. **VVL**

The pubic area is a highly sensitive place, so it's possible that a simple wax job may prove a painful experience. Sherri Shepherd, a comedian and former co-host from *The View*, did a YouTube video of her first bikini wax experience. She eschewed the prescribed numbing cream recommended to her as the newbie she was and concluded, "This is worse than having a baby!" Well, not really, I thought, but I felt her pain. If she had come to me first I would have insisted she spring for numbing cream an hour prior and an anti-inflammatory medication such as ibuprofen, and then I would have passed on the encouraging news that the discomfort of waxing eases over repeat sessions as the hair removed becomes weaker and grows more slowly. I would also advise any first timer to trim their pubic hair as short as possible before waxing. It also should be noted that skin irritation and ingrown hair can result after waxing, as can an increased chance of Staph infection around the hair follicle, called folliculitis, which may develop into abscesses if not treated properly. Although rare, labia tears can occur in an improperly executed wax job. Know your waxer, or get a referral. Whether you're a newbie or wax master, there are ways you can prepare for your waxing appointment.

Getting Ready for Your Bikini Wax Close-Up

* Shower before your appointment.
* Cut your pubic hair to no more than a quarter inch.
* Gently exfoliate your bikini line the night before.

* Find a qualified and reputable waxing facility! The extent of your satisfaction is directly related to your waxing professionals.
* And don't—DO NOT—shave between waxing sessions. Shaving chafes the skin and only serves to make the pubic hair sharper and coarser (and, thereby, more difficult to remove).

Laser Hair Removal

In this procedure, a laser is used to remove unwanted hair in the same way that lasers are often used to remove hair anywhere else on the body. Unlike waxing, however, laser treatments slow hair growth and, over continuous treatments, can result in permanent removal—although, there is no guarantee. Laser removal works best for light-skinned people with dark hair since the laser easily finds the hair against a lighter backdrop. A couple disadvantages to laser removal is that it can be costly and cause skin irritation, and, because of the possibility of skin discoloration, it works best only on certain skin and hair types. However, removing pubic hair with a laser can require longer stretches in between removal, thus causing fewer skin problems.

There's an interesting passage in Cameron Diaz's health and fitness book in the chapter "In Praise of Pubes." Apparently she is not a fan of permanent laser removal as she writes, "Personally, I think permanent laser hair removal sounds like a crazy idea. Forever? I know you may think you'll be wearing the same style of shoes forever and the same style of jeans forever, but you won't. The idea that vaginas are preferable in a hairless state is a pretty recent phenomenon, and all fads change, people."

Shaving (if You Must) Your Pubes

Yes, it is quick and easy to grab a razor and shave your pubic hair, but do heed a bit of advice if you chose this route.

Make certain to have a clean razor-blade, use shaving gel or cream with warm water, apply gentle pressure and use after-shave skin cream to keep the area hydrated and clean. Avoid products containing alcohol, and above all, never be in a rush when shaving.

Skin in the pubic hair area is especially sensitive and vulnerable to skin irritation—one of the reasons to use new blades is that old ones carry unwanted bacteria that can cause razor burns, bumps, acne, and other irritations to the skin and hair follicles. Although women (and men) love the look (and feel) of a freshly shaved vagina, unfortunately, that same desirable look and feel doesn't last too long with shaving. The hair that resurfaces tends to be thicker, pricklier and painful to the touch in its early stages of regrowth. Definitely not a sexy, feel-good experience for you or your partner.

Whether you chose the blade, laser, or wax for pubic hair removal, just make sure your skin is kept clean before and after. Using a loofah on the skin after any kind of hair removal helps to prevent ingrown hairs during regrowth. Non-fragrant soaps and lotions are also helpful in protecting this delicate area against acne, rashes, and other skin irritations.

If you're ready to tread further into sprucing up your vagina and pubic area, there are other creative avenues to explore, some of which are considered to be downright artistic. A few you may want to consider (or just *talk* about considering with some girlfriends at your next book club):

Vajazzling

What you get when you bedazzle the vagina: Vajazzling, a non-permanent, creative way of creating the glamorous vagina. A few years ago Jennifer Love Hewitt is believed to have helped coin this expression when she decorated her freshly waxed pubic area with Swarovski jewels—not to worry if you don't have the budget for these luxury-cut lead glass crystals; faux/plastic crystals are an inexpensive alternative. The process involves a paste application of the small ornaments around the pubic area after a full Brazilian. There are DIY kits, but the jury is still out on whether they're actually a cheaper alternative to using a vajazzling pro since even fake crystals have the potential to cut or mysteriously disappear in nearby orifices (yes, the vagina and anus) if improperly applied.

For those of you looking for a dazzling vagina makeover, this may be for you. **VVL**

Tattooing

Tattooing is an art form that has been around since the beginning of time, no matter what part of the body provides the canvas. A permanent tattoo is an everlasting piece of body art. If you're thinking of investing in such art do the research and give it as much thought as possible. You will carry this art with you for the rest of your life, so it is vital that you understand the process and risks of a tattoo, especially in the vaginal (and anal) area.

Tattoos are created with pigments that are inserted through pricks into the top layer of the skin. The tattoo artist uses a hand-held machine that employs multiple needles to deliver these tiny droplets of pigment or ink. The placement process can create a small amount of bleeding and pain. Typically, no anesthetics are used. **VVL**

A patient of mine, Rhonda, is a 27-year-old masseuse with the whole solar system tattooed on her body. Vividly rendered planets, moons, asteroids, and comets cover her chest, back, arms, and legs. Her body is a most fabulous canvas—although I do hope that she'll feel the same pull to the majesty of our planetary system in thirty years. When I told her that I was surprised she didn't have any tattoos on her vagina, she said that she preferred her clitoral hood **piercing** to ink, since the piercing made her sexual experiences more interesting and enjoyable. She said that she liked "the extra pressure the 'barbells' added" to her clit. **VVL**

Piercing

You name it, it can be pierced: ear, lip, bellybutton, nose... vagina. The risks and complications of piercing the vagina are the same as piercing any other part of your body, although the vagina is definitely a bit more sensitive to this particular process.

Certain risks are associated with piercing. These may include allergic reactions to nickel (a metal used in piercings), tearing or trauma from a piercing being caught or accidentally torn out, and, as is the same in tattooing: skin infections, skin problems such as scarring and keloids, and blood-borne disease from contaminated instruments.

If you chose to pierce your vagina or clitoral hood, make sure you consider the risks and complications and choose a reputable licensed body-piercing artist.

There are many other ways in which women may choose to decorate their vaginas. That said, I wanted to toss in a few "glamifying" methods that, thankfully, I've not yet seen in my practice (or personal life).

* Scarification, an art form in which a scar or keloid is intentionally created for ritual or decorative purposes.
* Subdermal implants, which are silicon implants placed directly under the skin, thereby creating a 3-D appearance.
* Skin stretching, which is typically seen in the earlobes (earlobe stretching). In earlobe piercing and stretching a hole is made and then stretched with a variety of objects such as rings and plugs. Vulvar Lip stretching has yet to catch on as a popular alternative.
* Branding, a form of scarification where a design is burned on the skin.

Vaginal Rejuvenation

Although controversial, there are some cosmetic vaginal surgeries which lay claims in providing a "designer vagina," "re-virgination," or "G-spot amplification" (rhymes not included). Kidding aside, there are doctors who may promote these surgeries but do be aware that they are not supported by the American College of Obstetrics and Gynecology and that they may present permanent complications such as pain with sex, scarring, and infection. Please get a second or third opinion with a reputable gynecologist before considering such a procedure.

To Glamify or Not to Glamify: Is That the Question?

Beauty is most certainly in the eye of the beholder, even when it comes to your vagina. To style or not to style your pubic hair, to pierce or tattoo, I would advise you to do what makes you feel best. What's important to *you*? Are you considering your partner's desires in lieu of your own?

What's most important is a clean, cared-for vagina. A glamorous vagina is one that is confident, and a confident vagina is, above all else, clean and healthy. Bedazzling can neither mask nor take the place of a well-tended V.

Please, don't commit to a tattoo or piercing unless you are mature enough to understand what's involved. And if you do decide to tattoo your vagina, promise me that you will not put your partner's name in ink. I know it's unromantic of me, but I'd be remiss if I didn't remind you that sixty percent of marriages end in divorce. Be creative, have fun, and ask yourself this: Would you, at sixty, want the same kitty art on your walls as you had when you were twelve? Just a thought.

Vagina bedazzled!

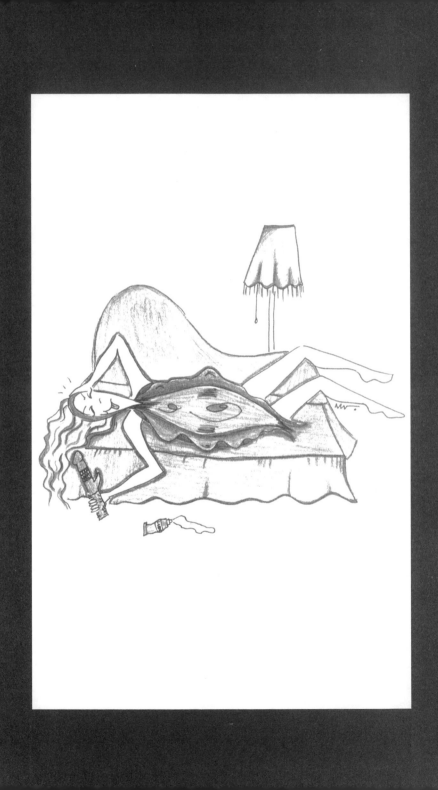

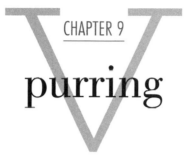

CHAPTER 9

purring

"Maybe you'll look me up. Maybe the first thing you find is this: Shannon Tweed Simmons is "...one of the most successful actresses of mainstream erotica.... Tweed lives with her husband Gene Simmons, co-lead singer of Kiss, and their two children.... [She] is also known for *Gene Simmons Family Jewels*, a TV reality show that portrayed the life of her family..."

So, let's get real…about sex and sexual satisfaction (known here as The Purring V). In real life nobody fucks half as long as they do in porn movies, and nobody screams out in ecstasy for that long either.

The reality of sex is a lot of silence (and grunting). The reality is that you have to identify your own route to pleasure on the map that is your own body, which will enable you to give your partner *direction*. The reality is that we all have our own secret fantasies, so find yours and keep it to yourself. Use your imagination, which ultimately means that this thing called *sexual satisfaction* is a lot up to you.

The reality is that with all the visual sex stuff at the fingertips of anyone with a cell phone, many are bound to feel, well, a little fucking insecure. I want to tell you not to be.

Nobody is perfect. No woman has tits like oranges (except maybe for about five minutes when they're sixteen).

Don't compare yourself to anyone. Not anyone. You do not need to live up to anyone else's standard.

Reality: Your partner especially doesn't want you to compare yourself to others. Think of it: If you compare yourself to some fleeting, unattainable idea of a sexual being, your partner will feel that they need to do the same. It's a recipe for insecurity, disappointment and, more importantly, no fun.

In short, get real. Know yourself. Know what satisfies you sexually, and be willing to communicate that to your partner. The bonus is that you'll naturally discover what satisfies the two of you together.

Your sexual life is not a show. It's not a movie. It's you and your imagination and self-knowledge and, with any luck, a partner in kind.

—Shannon Tweed Actress & Model

Anabella would be right out of Casting Central if the call was "Wanted: Seductive, gorgeous blond, late twenties." If this were the 1960s, men would stumble over themselves trying to be the first to light her cigarette. Add smarts and confidence to the mix, and you can understand Anabella's successful rise from the mailroom at William Morris Endeavor (WME), a powerhouse Los Angeles talent agency. At my practice, the few men in the vicinity may not stumble, but they (and women alike) do take notice of Anabella. I've seen it firsthand whenever she visits for her bi-yearly checkups. Yes, bi-yearly, which is not usually the norm. Admittedly, Anabella enjoys a very active sex life and understands the potential consequences of her large sexual appetite and multiple partners, so the regular visits quell her concerns about sexually transmitted infections (STIs). Early on in her visits Anabella wondered about her usual three to four orgasms during sex, since her friends seemed happy to have just one. She asked if she ought to be concerned. With a bit of a sigh (a little envy perhaps) I told her not to worry. She could rest assured that too many orgasms should be the least of her concerns.

Sex and Sexuality

Like a good auto mechanic who knows what each part under the hood of a car is called and what its function is, Anabella *knows* her vagina—knows her sweet spot and her vagina geography— which is important in understanding your sexuality. Though, truth be told, unless you *are* Anabella, you're probably content if you have one orgasm. Multiple orgasms are a *gift*—if only I could wrap them neatly in a box and sell them, I do believe I'd surpass the iPhone in sales—so if you're fortunate enough to experience multiple orgasms, consider yourself blessed. I'd venture to say that *one* orgasm in a sexual encounter is not only considered gratification enough, it's *the norm.*

The norm. What exactly is that?

Don't we all secretly wonder if we are **sexually normal**? But then what *is* sexually normal anyway? What does it mean? Does it even exist? I hear so many questions on this topic. They take the form of: *How often do women normally orgasm in vaginal intercourse? In oral sex? How often do women fake it? How often do women normally masturbate?* Think about it: Gather a cultural cross-section of a hundred "normal" women in a room. Will they look the same? Be of the same height and weight? Have the same morning routine, the same number of freckles and gray hairs? Of course not. And believe me, their vaginas will all have their own dimensions and personalities! According to a recent study from the University of Montreal, sexual desires and behaviors that are considered abnormal in psychiatry are actually *the norm*. So, unfortunately, there's no one-size-fits-all answer when it comes to sexual norm, but there is a way to help you understand your own *normal*—your own **sexuality**.

Sexuality is an important aspect of our wellbeing, and in a healthy romantic relationship it's as important as love and affection. Enjoyable sex is *learned*. Sure, there's instinct and maybe a dusting of magic involved, but you don't magically have an orgasm without having an active role in making it happen. You and your partner have to acknowledge each other's likes and dislikes, and *learn* how to satisfy each other. Open and honest conversations are necessary to make the sexual experience optimal for both of you, whether you have multiple partners or self-esteem to spare.

For women, the sexual experience can be broken down into four parts: desire, arousal, vaginal lubrication, and orgasm. I know you've heard it before, but it can't be overstated; your largest and most important sex organ is your *mind*. It's what makes all the parts come together in what can (and should) be a sublimely satisfying experience.

The Big O

What exactly is an orgasm (aside from purveyor of pleasure and satisfaction)? Medically speaking, it's a physical reflex, typically a pleasurable one—see, I told you—that occurs when muscles tighten during sexual arousal and then relax, thereby returning the body to its pre-arousal state.

Women achieve sexual pleasure primarily from the stimulation of the **clitoris,** a highly sensitive part of a woman's anatomy composed of millions of nerve endings similar to that of the penis. When your clitoris is touched, caressed, rubbed or stroked (with varying degrees of pressure) you may become sexually aroused, which can ultimately lead to orgasm. With sexual arousal, there is an increased blood flow to the genitals and the tensing of muscles throughout the body, *particularly* in the genitals. *Orgasm* reverses this process and returns your body to its pre-arousal state through a series of rhythmic contractions. Those contractions are felt in the vagina, uterus, anus, and pelvic floor. It's up to you to figure out what feels good, what degree of touch and exploration is most satisfying, and where, exactly, that elusive **G-spot** is hiding.

With that in mind, **masturbation** is the perfect way for you to get in touch with your own sexual pleasure by taking matters into your own hand, literally and figuratively.

A Magic Wand

Terri swears by hers. Although she's one of the most selfless and hardworking women I know, she's no Disney fairy godmother. Terri's "wand" is a vibrator from the popular sex toyshop goodvibrations.com, and Terri herself is a 39-year-old teacher in South Central Los Angeles who works mostly with kids that live in poverty—kids who likely live with one parent or an aunt or grandmother subbing as parent. A vivacious sparkplug of a gal, Terri has been single by choice and happy in her life for the ten years she's been my patient. She's a staunch joiner of every 5K run and 20K walk for a good cause and a collector of sponsors in raising funds to find the cure for everything from childhood leukemia to Alzheimer's. Over the years I've asked her variations of the same two questions: Do you have any new partners? Do you want kids of your own? She usually laughs long and hard. "Doctor Sherry, I have plenty of kids to love each and every day, and my current and only partner is 'Magic Monty,'" she says, referring to her magic wand. "He's the perfect partner—can't give me any STDs, doesn't give me shit, doesn't complain, doesn't leave any clothes on the floor, and gives me multiple orgasms...daily!"

Who am I to argue?

Obviously, you need not be single and uninterested in being with a partner, but Terri is certainly an example of a woman who has taken her sexual satisfaction into her own hands.

Taking the time to get in the mood and set up a relaxing environment can help to make your solo experience a success. Fingers, hands, lubricants, sex toys, porn, and fantasy are means to discovering your pleasure spots. For women, the average time to reach orgasm during masturbation is less than four minutes. For men, it's two to three minutes—which does nothing to disprove the theory that "men are easier." Maybe it's because we women have to satisfy the nerve endings from our vaginas all the way up to our brains! Just a little food for thought.

Helping the V Purr with a Partner

Ready, set, choose your positions! During sexual intercourse it's true that some positions are better than others in allowing the clitoris to be effectively stimulated. If you are on top during sex—a position known as the cowgirl position, with or without the cowboy hat—there's a better chance of your clitoris being stimulated than if you are in the missionary position. Similarly, if your partner enters from behind, they can simultaneously caress your clitoris. Experiment with your partner to find which position delivers the best results, and be patient. Statistics show that during foreplay and vaginal intercourse, the average time for women to reach orgasm is ten to twenty minutes; for men, seven to fourteen minutes overall, with an average of two to three minutes after beginning intercourse.

Vibrators and other sex toys are as helpful in achieving orgasm with a partner as they are in "solo" play. Go ahead, play, explore what feels good for you and have fun.

Is Orgasm Always the Goal?

Look, for some women, not achieving an orgasm during sexual activity is fine and acceptable. To these women, the closeness, touching, cuddling, kissing, and sharing of affection is more important than the actual orgasm. Other women may feel that if they don't have an orgasm they have a sexual problem or an **orgasmic disorder.**

A true orgasmic disorder is more likely the case for a woman who has *never* had an orgasm from any sexual contact or for one who may have had orgasms in the past but is no longer able to have them, despite being aroused in a healthy way—with age, orgasms may diminish somewhat in intensity, but they don't have to disappear. Causes of an orgasmic disorder include poor body image, fear of losing control, and a mistrust of one's partner. These factors can certainly hinder sexual arousal.

The physical *and* emotional changes that occur in the body because of sexual stimulation result in sexual arousal.

When you are aroused, not only does your heart rate and breathing increase, your nipples, labia, and clitoris fill with blood and become more sensitive, while your vagina naturally lubricates and expands. Arousal problems can be triggered by substance abuse involving smoking, alcohol or drugs, all of which affect the body in their own ways. If you can rule those factors out, there are ways to **increase your sexual arousal**:

* Increase time spent with foreplay.
* Use a vaginal lubricant such as KY and extra virgin coconut oil for vaginal dryness.
* Kegels! Come back to the K's. Kegel exercises help contract and relax pelvic muscles.
* Avoid tobacco. It restricts blood flow to the vagina.
* Experiment with sex toys.
* Use mental imagery and fantasy.

Of equal, if not greater importance is **sexual desire**. There are ways to improve that as well, such as:

* Focus more on intimacy and less on sexual intercourse.
* Address and try to resolve conflicts in your relationship. These conflicts may include stress or misunderstanding about sex or issues *outside* of sex— finances, kids, job insecurities—that are affecting you and your partner.
* Make time for sexual activity and focus less on sexual intercourse.
* Become more knowledgeable about sexual skills. Experiment.

If you happen to be in the process of learning the *art of orgasm*, and especially for those of you attempting to achieve multiple orgasms, you may find that you are experiencing an *ejaculatory* orgasm. This *once mythical* phenomenon regularly occurs in ten percent of women. Stimulation of the G-spot and clitoris in just the right way can actually cause an expulsion of fluid from your urethra, fluid that comes from the glands surrounding the urethra, resulting in—voila!—ejaculation.

The expectation of sexual satisfaction from one's partner is now the norm rather than the exception, but in order to let your partner know what feels good, you, yourself, must first know.

The Norm, in Conclusion

There really is no true definition of a *normal sex life*, especially now that women are, more than ever, becoming sexually empowered. If you are happy with your sexual experiences and the frequency of your orgasm, even if you don't have one every time, then that's *your* normal. What is normal for you may not be normal for your girlfriends, your sister, or (*gasp*) your mother.

What I would hope is that with each generation there are less and less sexual inhibitions and neuroses in the bedroom. Women must take the lead with intimacy. In doing so, not only will it become practice, it will lead to emotional and sexual confidence, which then leads to successful sexual relationships. Get comfortable with your body, your vagina, your clitoris. Find your sweet spot. Be the mechanic of your own body in order to have a lifetime of a Purring V.

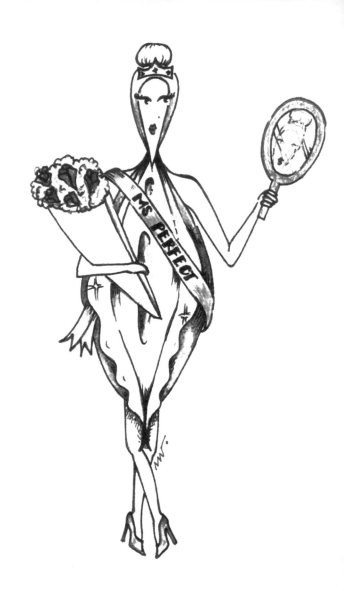

CHAPTER TEN

perfect

      As a kid, my parents would drive me all around Los Angeles to auditions. Since we lived in the OC—Orange County—that made for *long* car rides on the 405 Freeway. Needless to say, I spent a lot of time with my mom and dad—and you know how *helpful* parents can try to be when they have you trapped in a car during a long trip. Some of their advice went in one ear and out the other, but other words of wisdom stuck with me. What I do remember is how my parents always reminded me to be myself, to work hard and have fun, and to be grateful, kind, and respectful. I do try to be all those things, still.

      I like having a good time, laughing, playing practical jokes, and hanging out with my friends and family. The truth is I feel more comfortable in a pair of jeans, a tee shirt, a pair of old Converse sneakers and a black leather jacket than I do in dresses and heels. I admit it: I love being comfortable, relaxed, and makeup-free. There are always people who will rush to criticize you and make you feel badly about yourself, but because my parents helped instill confidence in me, I feel like a pretty normal person and I've learned to love my body, imperfections and all. You have to be comfortable in your own skin, which is something that Dr. Sherry has reminded me as well.

Dr. Sherry is my gynecologist. She has been taking care of me since I was nineteen, when I arrived for my first Pap smear. Let's face it, a Pap smear is not something you look forward to, but Dr. Sherry made an uncomfortable experience not so bad. In fact, because I have such a great relationship with Dr. Sherry—who never minds that I drag along my BFF Haley (who is also her patient!) so that we can laugh our way through the entire exam—I actually look forward to my yearly visits!

Every woman needs to find a gynecologist they feel comfortable with, especially one they can ask those really embarrassing questions— you know the ones I'm talking about. I am so glad to introduce the Perfect V chapter, because to me the Perfect V is a healthy V, which means yearly checkups and conversations about the importance of safe sex.

My mom told me that the first step to self-confidence was to feel positive about my body. I can still hear her say to me, "When you smile, you are beautiful." I think smiling shows the world that you believe you're beautiful regardless of what others may think. It's exactly like "You are what you think."

I am so lucky to have fallen into acting, and I *really* appreciate all my amazing fans. If I can send a positive message to teens and young women about their bodies, it would be: *Love your perfect V. Love your body no matter the size or shape. Don't allow anyone to judge your lady parts, especially your pretty little V!*

—**Ashley Benson** Actress & Model

Perfect V

Out of the blue, Lauren, a smart and adorable 21-year-old patient of mine, thinks the lips of her vagina are too big. Her older boyfriend of four months, Jake, apparently made comments about her plus-size vaginal lips, telling her, "You don't have a sexy cooch"—this after Lauren had her clit pierced at Jake's request. I did Lauren's first gynecological exam and Pap smear when she was seventeen, and I can't help think about how she graduated in the top tenth percentile of her high school, earned a black belt in Tae Kwon Do and received a full scholarship to the University of Pennsylvania, but ended up attending the local city college so she wouldn't leave her single mom alone. When I think of this, I want to give Jake more than a piece of my mind, since Lauren tearfully went on about how ashamed she felt. She asked how she could get "the perfect vagina." I hugged her and reassured her that she was perfect in every way, especially her vagina. Having three sons who hated it when I started talking about the vagina made me mother Lauren more than usual. The time I spent giving Lauren straight talk about what a "perfect" vagina really looked like felt essential to her empowerment as a strong, healthy, "perfect" woman.

You know the saying, "No two snowflakes are exactly alike?" Well, the expression could just as easily refer to vaginas. There is no one right way for a vagina to look, meaning that there's no such thing as a perfect one. If anyone should know that, it's an OB-GYN who's been seeing patients and their vaginas for nearly three decades.

The labia, or lips—which is where most of the issues are for the majority of female patients—vary from person to person. In fact, even the separate parts of the same vagina are not exactly the same. Just as our two eyes are not identical, nor our ears or breasts, our two lips are not identical, nor are they symmetrical to each other. This is considered to be completely normal; different is normal. I'll tell you (in short) what I told Lauren: The only qualities that make a vagina "perfect" are good health and confidence.

And yet...

These days, social media allows all of us to compare ourselves to others in every way possible, including our vaginas. So I wasn't all that surprised when another of my young patients—one a few years younger than Lauren—asked if I thought her lips were "abnormally large." She went on to say her boyfriend (again with the "expert" boyfriend) told her that her lips were too big compared to others he'd seen. When I asked her who the "others" were, it turned out they were the women on the porn sites he visited. Sadly, I wasn't at all shocked to hear this, because, unfortunately, he's the norm, not the exception.

Dr. Gail Dines—http://gaildines.com—is a professor of sociology, modern day hero and a leading anti-porn feminist committed to tying down the "porn monster that has taught our girls to hypersexualize and pornify themselves." As founder of Culture Reframed, the first health promotion effort to recognize and address pornography as the public health crisis of the digital age, Dr. Dines is on a mission to provide education and support to promote healthy child and youth development, relationships, and sexuality. If she has her way, this type of education will be as standard in public school systems as, say, student driving and drinking prevention programs were when I attended public school.

There's no denying it. Porn is everywhere. Dr. Dines puts a perspective on this issue of accessibility of porn when she tells us, "Porn sites get more visitors each month then Netflix, Amazon, and Twitter combined." A recent statistic found that seventy percent of children ages eight to eighteen report having unintentionally stumbled across pornography online. The average age for a child to be exposed to pornography is now eleven years old. This means that our children are often "learning" about "normal" sexual behavior and physical appearance from the likes of Jenna Jameson and John Holmes. Many women (and men) now expect, even want, all vaginas to look like Jenna's docs. Girls and guys alike visit porn and other sexually graphic web sites, and not just to get off, but also to see what the perfect vagina and the ideal penis look like.

As a result of social media, some women have been made to feel vagina insecurity. And I'm not just seeing this in patients, either, although it's definitely something that comes up regularly in my examining room. It's everywhere. An Internet search of the word "vagina" brings up a variety of links, many leading to everyday women showing off their vaginas: You Tube videos of women talking about vaginal rejuvenation, websites devoted to discussing and examining anything vagina related, and, of course, porn sites. These are the reference points that young women—women of all ages, really—now use when seeking the ideal of the perfect vagina. Adolescent boys are having the same issues regarding the size and length of their penises, even though, like vaginas, no two penises or scrotums are the same.

This is where I come in—with my agenda of vagina empowerment! I want to reduce your anxiety and help you have more realistic expectations about what's normal by giving you an accurate view of the vagina in general. Believe me, the perfect vagina is actually a medical norm and not an aesthetic ideal.

Here is an overview of what normal anatomy looks like for the female external genitalia.

As Close to Perfect As Perfect Gets

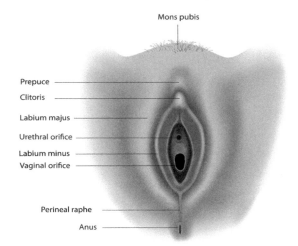

What we think of as the vagina actually includes the outer labia majora (lips), inner labia minora (lips), clitoris (clit), clitoral hood, opening to the urethra and opening to the vagina. You need to get to know and love all parts of this fascinating area of your body. Know what *your* "normal" is so you will know when something is not normal or when a potential problem arises. **VVL**

Our Version of Perfect

Much as women have always compared their bodies and breasts to models and movie stars, now the vagina is up for inspection. I hear comments like: "My lips are too big," "too bumpy," "too dark," "too uneven," "too *in the way*." Or: "My boyfriend/girlfriend tells me my labia are not pretty," or "not sexy."

Perfect V

More and more, my patients are asking me what the perfect vagina looks like and how they can get one. Women of all ages, including adolescents, are now aware of cosmetic genital procedures that vow to make the vagina beautiful, even perfect. I get a lot of inquiries about these alterations and what they can and can't do.

While my goal is to care for my patients and make their lives better, from their health and wellbeing to their level of self esteem and sexual pleasure, I sometimes have to dole out some tough love when it comes to their quest for the perfect vagina. If having surgery will make a patient feel happier and more confident, I can absolutely see the benefit. And yet, I always caution her to really think her decision through before she does anything drastic. I ask my patients to honestly consider the following:

"Is this absolutely necessary?"

"What does the perfect vagina really look like anyhow?"

"Does Jenna Jameson have the perfect vagina? Really?"

"How will my life (and sex life) be improved by having a different vagina?"

Even minor surgery can lead to complications. And if this quest is undertaken for the wrong reasons, or with unrealistic expectations, even a positive outcome can be disappointing. I think it's important to remember that the media's perception of genital anatomy is often not representative of the general population. Real indications that something is actually wrong with your vagina include discomfort, pain, itching, odor, or discharge. Short of that, the issue you're obsessing about might just be in your mind. So, before you do anything cosmetic and permanent, think about it, talk to your doctor, talk to your friends—have a long, hard, compassionate look at your vagina. Know what you're really dealing with before you embark on a drastic plan. In other words, educate yourself.

There Is No Perfect. But There Is Normal.

The Abnormal V

While a wide range of variety is the norm when it comes to vaginas, there are women out there who do have abnormal labia. But, again, this has nothing to do with aesthetics. For most, there's no denying that something isn't quite right. The most common symptom is the need to fold up their labia and push them into their vaginas in order to reduce the appearance of excess tissue or a bulge in their underwear or bathing suits. Other symptoms include labial pain, swelling, irritation, poor hygiene, and interference with athletics or sexual activity. Oversized or enlarged labia can impact athletics, such as running, bicycling, horseback riding, and swimming. Surgical procedures are available to improve these symptoms, as well as the appearance of the vagina. **VVL**

Vagina Envy

When they do occur, noticeably enlarged labia are not just an aesthetic issue, especially during adolescence. Young girls with vaginas that look different are often self-conscious and reluctant to undress in front of their peers. Psychological problems can occur, including severe emotional distress, depression, and anxiety. In these instances, surgery can be a great solution.

When Sophia, a shy, conscientious 16-year-old high school junior came in for her first gynecological exam, she asked her mom—who was also my longtime patient—to wait in the lobby. Her independence really impressed me. Sophia talked about school, how awesome Claire Danes is in *Homeland*, and her two dogs, Scottie and Jack. As she began talking about her love of the water and making the swim team, she became so nervous that she started to chew on her hair. She finally admitted that she didn't feel comfortable changing into her bathing suit with her teammates. In a whisper, she asked, "Is it normal to have to tuck my lips into my vagina before I go swimming?" She went on to say that before swim practice or meets she went into a bathroom stall and folded her lips up so they wouldn't bulge out of her bathing suit.

When I examined Sophia, her labia on the right side was, in fact, six inches longer than on the left side, and the difference was quite noticeable. We discussed surgical options, which, in Sophia's case, could work wonders for her self-esteem and feeling of well-being. **VVL**

The Benefits of Surgery

The primary procedure to repair such abnormal labia is called labiaplasty. A trained plastic surgeon or gynecologist can perform this simple outpatient procedure, and the results can be life changing. As with any surgery, however, complications can occur. The most commonly seen side-effect of this procedure is painful scarring that can lead to discomfort during sex. As always, it's important to have a candid talk with your doctor and maintain realistic expectations.

The Clit and Nothing But the Clit

Striding down the hallway to my office, Chloe—a vibrant, confident, plus-sized 43-year-old longtime patient—works her three-inch heels and skin-tight animal-print dresses as if she's on a fashion runway. Every time she visits, she brings a five-pound box of See's candy (nuts and chews—my favorite), and makes sure everyone gets a chocolate and a big squeeze. As soon as Chloe sees my nurse, she shouts out her trademark greeting, "Hey, girl, hey!" Once during an exam, Chloe asked me if more women have an innie or an outie clit. She then told me about her friend Sasha, who claimed to have a giant clit. She admitted that they'd recently played that old school yard game: If you show me yours, I'll show you mine, because Chloe was sure that her friend was "making this shit up." Chloe told me, "Sure enough, Sasha's clit was like a small penis! If I hadn't seen it with my own two eyes, I would not have believed it." She wondered if her friend's orgasms were bigger; since her clit was triple the size of Chloe's. I have to say that honest and inquisitive conversations like this are especially engaging as a doctor, which is why Chloe is one of my favorite patients.

In medical terms, the clitoris is actually referred to as a phallus, just like a penis is. That's where the similarities stop, though. The normal size for a clitoris is 5 mm in length. With 8,000 highly sensitive nerve endings, its main—really, its only function—is to give pleasure. Meanwhile, the penis only has 4,000 nerve endings. However, size doesn't have anything to do with pleasure. As I told Chloe, a bigger clitoris does not mean a more intense orgasm, nor does a smaller clitoris mean any less pleasure. So worry not.

Consistent with this chapter's theme, no two clitorises look the same, just as the vaginas in which they reside are all different. Some are thinner, wider, shorter, or longer than others. There are some abnormally enlarged clitorises out there, like one that measured twenty mm (or five times the normal size!) and, on arousal, measured thirty mm. Known as clitoromegaly, this condition can be due to hormones, medications, congenital malformation, or other unknown causes. In such cases, surgery is performed to correct the abnormal enlargement. But, as with vaginas, most differences in size and shape are considered totally normal, and if we change our mindsets, may be considered beautiful in their variations.

Vaginal "Rejuvenation"

Our current cultural obsession with the perfect vagina is causing a lot of unfounded promises to be made out there, including vaginal "rejuvenation," cosmetic vaginal surgeries promising to create a "designer vagina," "re-virgination," or "G-spot amplification." While some doctors do promote and recommend these procedures, they are very controversial. Be aware that these surgeries are not supported by the American College of Obstetrics and Gynecology, and they can result in permanent complications that could affect sexual sensation or cause scarring, infection, or pain with sex. Always get a second or third opinion from a reputable gynecologist before considering a procedure you may regret in the future.

When another young patient of mine, Sandy, asked me why women wanted the perfect V, I could only share with her my philosophies of life. Sandy came in for a routine Pap and STI testing, which I performed, but I also talked to her as though I were talking to my own kids. I explained that those who wanted the perfect V—who wanted the perfect *anything*—had personal struggles, and that their quest really reflected a need to be flawless...which is not only unrealistic, it is impossible to achieve. People are not meant to be perfect. In fact, those who strive for perfection are often masking their own insecurities and vulnerabilities. I told Sandy the same thing that I tell the majority of my patients, that she already had the perfect V. There will always be unrealistic notions of "perfection," but you mustn't take those notions to heart. If you do, you'll ultimately be crushingly disappointed...and unhappy. **VVL**

Maybe, rather than doing anything drastic, consider joining the vagina revolution. Choose to love and empower your vagina as it is now. It's beautiful and powerful, just the way it is, just like you.

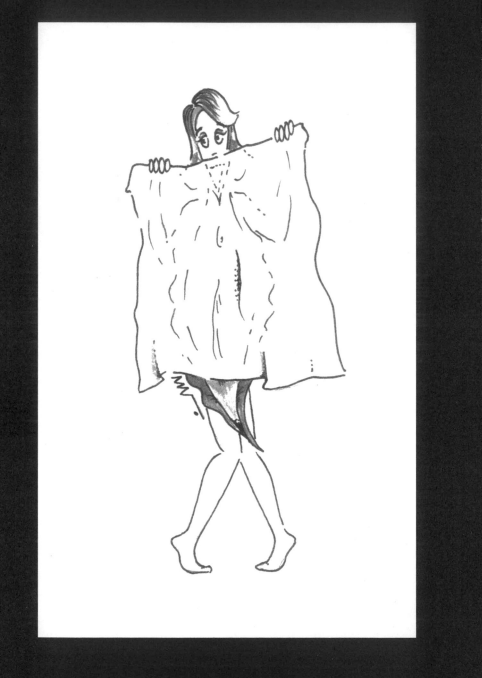

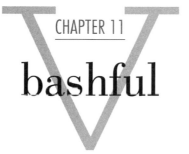

CHAPTER 11

bashful

"I want to come at this straight. I want to bring my own baggage and unpack it in front of you.

I am one of the Bashful Bunch — or at least I'm still working my way out of membership in the group. To many of my friends, I am a walking contradiction. I appear extroverted and at ease with myself, which for the most part I am. I have taught women's studies in college and have spent the better part of the last decade facilitating women's groups and writing books on women's empowerment. Yet, I still revert to the early conditioning of my Middle Eastern culture when it comes to matters of sex.

It was one autumn afternoon in the fourth grade when I asked my mom how babies were made. She was chopping basil and mint leaves in the kitchen and the smell of the fresh-cut herbs was permeating the house. I was standing next to her when I asked "the question." An awkward silence ensued. My mom didn't look up; she paused for a moment and then proceeded to chop the remaining bunch of green herbs scattered on the counter. When she was finished, she cleaned her hands on her apron, went to look out the window, and then turned and said, "When a husband and wife really want and love each other, babies are made." That was it. She then hurried out of sight. That, I can tell you, was the extent of my sex talk with my mom.

So, you could only imagine my utter bewilderment in sixth grade, when I took my first sex-education class in the United States. That same year many Iranians escaped the revolution in Iran and transplanted themselves in Los Angeles. In class, we Iranian girls kept our heads down and cast furtive glasses at each other in between sneak peaks at the slides projected on the classroom screen. In our culture, chastity and modesty were values central in raising "proper" girls, oftentimes to the point that we were estranged from our own sexuality and bodies.

In time I realized that there were many women from other walks of life with similar experiences. Because I was a young and approachable teacher, many freshman and sophomore college girls in my classes visited me during office hours to discuss personal matters as well as academic ones. One wary student confided that that her body consciousness held her back from intimacy, while another super-achieving student broke down in tears and shared that she had been hiding her pregnancy from friends and family. In my women's group, many shared their struggles to shake off shame and undo old inhibitions as they approached midlife.

It is true that all of us navigate this complex world according to the beliefs and values we have been raised with or hold close to our hearts. But, our individual baggage is never just ours alone. It belongs to the collective.

Bashful V

I believe that every woman should have the opportunity at some point in her life to set down and unpack her sexual baggage among those she trusts and respects. That is the first step to reclaiming our bodies, our health, our pleasure, and our wholeness as feminine beings.

It is because of that belief that I am grateful for the work that Dr. Sherry does every day. She has devoted her life to the female body—how to talk about it, protect it, and value it. In this book, Dr. Sherry ventures into topics about which most of us women are curious to know and understand but may be too embarrassed to verbalize. 99

—**Angella Nazarian** Author & International Speaker

Athletic and outgoing, Tammy is an attractive 23-year-old student at Boulder College. She drops in for her checkups during summer and Christmas breaks, always sure to remind me to check for STDs. Tammy's naturally inquisitive nature, combined with her major in Women's Studies, always make for lively and progressive conversations. She'd never been hesitant to ask anything about her body, until her last visit. As tears welled up in her eyes, she looked directly at me and confessed, "I have to ask you something, but it's completely embarrassing." I assured her that there was little chance of her embarrassing herself, especially in front of me. "Okay," she said, and then blurted out, "I don't think I've ever had an orgasm!" And the conversation began.

All of us are a product of our upbringing—parents, siblings, best friends, partners past and present—and, for some of us, our religion. Often times, what's forgotten in that upbringing is the encouragement to explore one's sexuality. Ironic, really, because *sexuality* is as part of our lives as eating and sleeping (the companion to this chapter is Purring V, but first, read on). The obvious solution to this omission is the pursuit of your own personal sexual revelations. It's time to take that bashful vagina in hand (literally) and lead the exploration.

Bashful V? I'm talking about the inability to have or ask for the sexual pleasure associated with vaginal stimulation. Whether you've never had an orgasm, or you have certain sexual or emotional issues that get in the way of intimacy, there are things you can do to acquaint your Bashful V with some fun.

Many women have a very difficult time achieving orgasm. Through the years I've met a number of women in their thirties, forties, and fifties who have never even *had* an orgasm. In fact, ten to twenty percent of all women have never experienced one. That information was certainly a shock to Tammy, although it did squelch her tears a bit in knowing that she wasn't alone, and that there was a *solution.*

Masturbation: Stigmas Need Not Apply!

First let me say that masturbation is a completely normal, common activity that is completely healthy! It is an act during which you touch or self-stimulate your genitals to achieve sexual arousal and pleasure, resulting in an orgasm...but, not always. A recent study revealed that 89% of women masturbate and 95% of men. Masturbation tends to be the very first sexual experience to bring on an orgasm for both sexes. Unfortunately, masturbation is a topic that is strictly off limits in some circles. The word alone can bring about embarrassment, insuring shame and anxiety around the very thought of it.

The Benefits of Masturbation
(or Why Have a Date with Rosey Palmer?)

* You will understand what makes you feel good so you may help your partner with a successful road map in bed.
* It's a sexual activity that's not only normal and healthy, it's pleasurable and safe.
* It's the perfect tension and stress reliever.
* It's a natural sleeping pill.
* It's a guaranteed way to avoid STIs and pregnancy.

Is Masturbation Ever Harmful?

* Rarely. Trauma to your lady parts, including the vagina, labia or clitoris is more likely when using objects not meant to be used inside the vagina.
* Certain cultures and religion deem masturbation a sin, which may make the act a shameful one, leading to great guilt and distress.
* Excessive masturbation that interferes with your daily life may cause anxiety.

The Clitoris: Ready for Its Close-up

It may (or may not) surprise you to learn that in a recent survey among young women ages 16–25, half could not find the vagina on a medical diagram. Not only could they not identify the diagramed V, sixty-five percent of those women were so embarrassed to say the word "vagina" they had to use slang terms in referring to it. A test group of university-aged women didn't fare much better in their vagina knowledge. One third of the group was unable to find the clitoris on a medial diagram. Clearly, if you can't find the clit, how are you going to seek enjoyment from it?

With its *8,000 highly sensitive nerve endings*, the main function of the clitoris is to give pleasure! Compare that to its male equivalent, the penis, which pales in comparison with a mere 4,000 nerve endings.

The clitoris is basically the female version of the penis. When stimulated, the clitoris becomes hard and grows to *three times its size*, in the same way that the penis does—however, the clitoris takes longer than the penis for that arousal, around ten to fifteen minutes longer. You can stimulate the clitoris with fingers, the tongue, or with the penis during vaginal intercourse, but remember that it is extremely delicate and needs a soft touch initially. Take time to figure out your personal preference. You may realize that after light stimulation, harder and stronger pressure is needed to reach orgasm. Incidentally, most women agree that the best stimulation of the clitoris comes from the tongue.

Now What?

Masturbation is a skill. It has to be learned, just as walking, running, singing, and brushing your teeth (although it's a bit more fun than flossing).

First, the **setting** must be right. Being in the mood and creating a relaxing environment will help make your experience a success. Get rid of distractions, turn off your cell phone, turn on relaxing music, clear your mind, focus, and empower yourself by taking control of your emotional, physical, and sexual needs.

Try using two fingers and a vaginal lubricant to gently stroke the area on and around the clitoris and clitoral hood.

Bashful V

You may start by touching your clit lightly at first, followed by harder and stronger pressure as it becomes stimulated and hard. This may take ten minutes to an hour. As the clit is stimulated, you can squeeze your butt cheeks together, which contracts your pelvic floor muscles—basically you're doing Kegels! The Kegel contractions can help you achieve an orgasm. As the pleasure builds in your clitoral area, it spreads throughout your body, affirming your methods.

As I talked about in the Purring V (Chapter 15) you may want to move onto lubricants with sex toys, porn and fantasy in finding how to bring yourself pleasure. One of the most popular vibrators is the "Original Magic Wand," sometimes referred to as the holy grail of vibrators. My only issue with this super-duper high-powered vibrator is that it has only 2 speeds—powerful and even more powerful—which makes the experience quick, intense and sometimes a bit overwhelming. The next generation of "OMW" has 4 speeds and gets the job done with a more modern look, feel and attitude. That said, my personal favorite is called the Inspire Vibrating Ultimate Wand by Calexotics, which has 10 speeds with varying intensities from gentle to vigorous, plus it's made from silicone, which feels really good on the vagina and clitoris. Other perks are that it's waterproof, rechargeable, and travel friendly, the perfect trifecta for your favorite vibrator!

What's important is that *you* know what feels good and what doesn't. Intimacy and sexual satisfaction are basic, instinctual human needs. Help your partner by verbalizing what feels good. In order to do that, you must be able to say it to yourself. Talk to a healthcare provider you trust if you feel you need help in talking with your partner.

Call it polishing the pearl, or beating the bishop; it doesn't matter. Make up your own private name for pleasuring yourself, as long as you realize that it's a normal and healthy pastime with proven health benefits. It's time for your Bashful V to take charge!

Masturbation Taboos

Magdalena and her husband, mother, grandmother, and five children arrived in Los Angeles from Mexico seven years ago. Like many immigrants, Magdalena and her husband wanted better opportunities for their children. A soft-spoken, tireless 42-year-old, Magdalena never neglected to bring her fabulous homemade tamales to the office for the entire staff. My weakness was for her homemade habanero salsa, which she'd slip to me in a large Tupperware bowl. Magdalena spoke in Spanglish, a version of English and Spanish combined, which I could mostly understand. On this particular visit she said to me, "Yo nunca he tenido un orgasm." Well, I knew enough Spanish to know that she was saying that she'd never had an orgasm. Ironically, her next sentence was in perfect English: "Can you help me find a way to have one?" I was able to find out that she'd never touched herself, meaning that she had never masturbated.

Attitudes regarding sex, sexuality and gender vary greatly between different cultures and religions. Certain sexual practices, traditions, and taboos are passed down through generations, leaving little to the cause of female pleasure or imagination. As in the case of a devout Catholic like Magdalena, sex (and sexual pleasure, if there is any) is tied only to procreation. In most cultures around the world, the idea that women might feel or want sexual pleasure is not even entertained.

Why Am I Not Enjoying Sex?

For some women, finding and/or enjoying sexual intimacy and sex is difficult, if not impossible. Research suggests that forty-three percent of women report some degree of difficulty and twelve percent attribute their sexual difficulties to personal distress. Unfortunately, sexual problems worsen with age, peaking in women forty-five to sixty-four. For many of these women, the problems of sexual dysfunction are treatable, which is why (again) it is so important for women to share their feelings and concerns with a healthcare provider.

There are five main problems under the umbrella of **Female Sexual Dysfunction (FSD)**:

* Low libido or Hypoactive Sexual Desire Disorder (HSDD), a condition signified by a disinterest in having sex, is the most common cause of a low desire in women.
* Painful sex, which may stem from pain or burning during sex due to vaginal dryness or vaginal atrophy due to menopause (a time when estrogen is no longer around to hydrate the vaginal tissue).
* Difficulty in becoming sexually aroused, conveniently termed Sexual Arousal Disorder.
* Aversion to sex, a problem that tends to be associated with a history of sexual abuse.
* Inability to achieve orgasm.

Understanding the cause of the sexual dysfunction is the most important step in optimizing a **treatment plan.**

Relationship counseling, stress reduction, sex therapy, or a weekend away with your partner without the kids may be all that's needed to get you back on track.

Unfortunately, there has been a history of "gender injustice" in the bedroom. Women have long been ignored when it comes to finding solutions to sexual dysfunction. If there were a scoreboard it would read 26 to 0 for men! In short, there are *twenty-six* approved medications for male erectile dysfunction and *zero* for women. Clearly, little attention has been paid to the sexual concerns of women, other than those concerns that involve procreation. The FDA claims that it wants to approve medications for female sexual dysfunction, but they are waiting for ones with minimal side effects, substantial health benefits, and unlikely potential for misuse—a tall order indeed, especially for the estimated sixteen million women in the U.S. who suffer from a lack of libido.

Hypoactive sexual disorder, the most common female sexual dysfunction, is characterized by a complete absence of sexual desire. For the sixteen million women who suffer from this disorder, the factors involved may vary since sexual desire in women is much more complicated than it is for men. Unlike men, women's sexual desire, excitement, and energy tend to begin in that great organ *above the shoulders*, rather than the one *below the waist*. The daily stresses of work, money, children, relationships, and diminished energy are common issues contributing to low libido in women. Other causes may be depression, anxiety, lack of privacy, medication side effects, medical conditions such as endometriosis or arthritis, menopausal symptoms such as a dry vagina, or a history of physical or sexual abuse. It's not a myth after all that women are more *complicated* than men.

Bashful V

Is Help On the Way?

Flibanserin, a drug commonly known as **Addyi**, is the first official drug to show some benefit in improving sexual satisfaction in premenopausal women, although it is not without controversy.

While women on Addyi have showed a slight (10%) improvement in the frequency of satisfying sexual encounters and an increase in their desire for sex, Addyi critics suggest that "flawed and inaccurate data was presented to promote the doctors own agenda." The FDA still has serious concerns about the *side effects* of Addyi, which include drowsiness, fainting, and low blood pressure, all of which are exacerbated with medications such as *antidepressants* and *alcohol*—which means that Addyi and Happy Hour definitely don't mix. As with any medication, you must discuss with your physician whether you're an appropriate candidate for this particular drug. Despite the jury still being out, many experts don't think the studies support the benefits of using Addyi.

Testosterone is another treatment alternative that may help with low libido. Side effects of excessive use of this potent, well-known hormone include acne, facial hair growth, aggressive behavior, and voice changes. It is primarily recommended for postmenopausal women.

An FDA-approved electrical stimulator known as the **EROS device** can help women achieve an orgasm, although a good vibrator from your favorite sex shop will be far less costly and may well achieve the same goal.

Menopausal women may benefit from vaginal estrogen, vaginal DHEA or Osphena, an FDA-approved, non-hormonal oral treatment for painful intercourse, as Addyi is *not* recommended for postmenopausal women. (Studies didn't support its effectiveness for this particular group.) The Mona Lisa laser is an exciting new treatment for vaginal dryness caused by menopause that restores the collagen, elastin, and blood flow of the vagina.

Women simply want the same attention in sexual health and responsiveness from the medical community as men have had. With that in mind, the FDA is finally showing support for the challenges faced in female sexual health. Whether you choose a medical alternative, a little self-love in the afternoon, or a romantic weekend without electronics or distractions, the choice should be yours.

"Yes-Yes-Yes!"...Who Is Faking It?

Orgasm is obvious, right? In crossing the orgasmic finish line, your male partner ejaculates, and, if you're a woman, you may tend towards something more, well, verbal. It's true: women *are*, for the most part, more verbal than men in sex—as well as in a whole host of other circumstances. According to a large study by Charlene Muehlenhard, a professor of clinical psychology at the University of Kansas in Lawrence, women tend to rely on more obvious signs and vocalizations to alert their partner of "mission accomplished." Muehlenhard also says that studies done since the 70s repeatedly show, on average, heterosexual women fake their orgasms 59% of the time during vaginal sex. Similar studies find the same percentage fake orgasms during oral sex, too.

Dr. Erin Cooper, a clinical psychologist at Temple University, found in a study on a college campus that the main reasons women fake orgasm is "out of concern for a partner's feeling, fear of negative emotions associated with the sexual

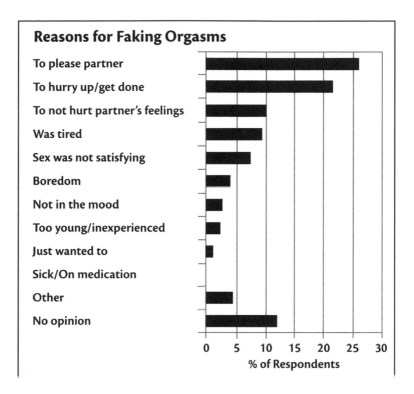

Reasons for Faking Orgasms

- To please partner
- To hurry up/get done
- To not hurt partner's feelings
- Was tired
- Sex was not satisfying
- Boredom
- Not in the mood
- Too young/inexperienced
- Just wanted to
- Sick/On medication
- Other
- No opinion

0   5   10   15   20   25   30
% of Respondents

experience, sexual insecurity about their own dysfunction, concerns about being abnormal, to end sex and [interestingly enough] to increase their own sexual arousal." ABC News put the graph above together to show all the reasons why women fake their orgasms.

A study from the *Journal of Sex Research* found that women having lesbian sex experience higher rates of orgasm than their straight counterparts, that they have sex more often, and that they have higher levels of sexual satisfaction. Sort of makes sense since lesbians are more in touch and acquainted with other women's bodies, making navigation easier. But, ladies, get ready for this tidbit: researchers also discovered that 24% of men fake *their* orgasms! What was *their* main reason for faking it? The desire to get sex over with!

If you desire real sexual satisfaction but find yourself faking orgasms more often than not, especially with a partner you are truly interested in, it's best to be open about your issues and consider seeking professional help. Bashful V does not need to fake it anymore.

It's funny, when you think men literally hold their penises *at least* a couple times a day in the average course of peeing. They know exactly what their sex organ feels and looks like. Not so much for women because of the vagina's internal existence, which means that we have to make a concerted effort to get to know our vaginas. In knowing, we also discover what feels good.

You are the person in charge of your vagina and clitoris. First and foremost, get to know your female parts intimately. Understanding your sexual response is a necessary health and wellness skill. Make mastery of that skill a priority. You are the one to lead yourself to your own sexual freedom and satisfaction. Investigate, masturbate, give your vagina the attention it needs and deserves. After all, you have the power to avoid a Bashful V!

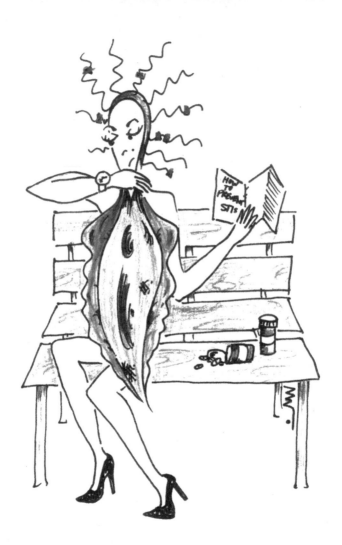

CHAPTER 12

benched

"My father, Vidal Sassoon, was not only an icon in the beauty industry, he left a legacy of an unwavering sense of humanity, and he made a difference in so many people's lives. He gave me the gifts of strength, creativity, compassion, and love. He would say, "My darling Eden, she is the most like me."

My father passed away five years ago when I was thirty-eight, at a point when I still felt very much like a little girl. Only then did I realize it was time for me to grow up.

Dr. Sherry has been taking care of me since I was eighteen. She saw me through all the bad decisions and mistakes I made, especially concerning the care of my vagina. My V was benched a couple of times in my early adulthood, but those days are way behind me. Alcohol, smoking, and a general disrespect of my body were bad habits that I overcame as I arrived at my current chosen path, a path of sobriety, healthy eating, regular exercise, and being in tune with my heart and soul.

She-ology

If you've ever had a Benched V, my advice to you is to learn from it, and then don't let it happen again! I would leave you with one of my most cherished mantras: This Too Shall Pass. Learn from your painful experiences, take care of yourself, respect yourself, and take pride in your health and who you are.

At forty-three I am now a single, sober mother who is not afraid to share the good and bad stories of a life well lived or the horror stories of how alcohol made me do things that I am not proud of.

Which brings me back to my father. He was my mentor, my hero, the person I most aspired to be. Shortly before he died, he asked me, 'What are you going to do with your life, with yourself?'

I know now with great clarity that I want to be present, be in the moment, and to make a difference each and every day. Having fought off my own personal demons and come out on the other side, I am proud to say that I am finally a true reflection of my father. What I would hope for all women is that they, too, find their joy and their passion for their health, beauty, and fitness.

Regarding that Benched V: Take the time and care to make that V a *joyous* one instead! 99

—Eden Sassoon Entrepreneur, Reality TV Personality

Debbie is a gregarious 22-year-old sparkplug of a gal. A third year student at Pepperdine, a university near Malibu overlooking the Pacific Ocean, Debbie is studying art history and economics with the same fervor (perhaps obsession) she has for everything natural and environmentally friendly. Unfortunately, that avoidance of things she deems "unnatural" includes anything "prescription." Instead of using the pill as contraception, Debbie optioned for a special **fertility monitor** from the UK that, as she said, "worked perfectly at avoiding pregnancy if used backwards!"—which meant that she avoided sex when the monitor signaled she was ovulating. She proudly dismissed the Gardasil vaccine claiming she "didn't want to be another statistic of a vaccine failure." Debbie often suffered from vaginal itching and a thick, curdled discharge—along with other telltale signs of yeast infection. She swore by her own homemade concoction to cure the symptoms, "Grandma Sadie's yogurt remedy," but she was in my office because the remedy had not provided any recent relief. Was I surprised? Maybe not so much.

Your very sensitive V can be benched for a number of reasons. I say "benched" because there are many vaginal infections ranging from mild to severe that can keep you from sex, sports, a comfortable day at the office, or a healthy life! As with my advice in Cranky V (Chapter 13), it takes a visit to your healthcare provider to diagnose and treat the Benched V. You would be amazed by the number of women I see who have unknowingly contracted Chlamydia or Gonorrhea or who don't realize they're in the midst of the most common of vaginal infections, a **yeast infection** (which happens when bad bacteria in the vagina outnumber the good). Sometimes a round of **antibiotics** for a sinus infection is enough to set off this most simple and prevalent of infections.

The good bacteria that protect the vagina can also be disrupted by a number of environmental, physical, and stress-related factors. Not surprisingly, thirty percent of women will develop some **inflammation** of the vagina, for which the medical term is **vaginitis**.

(Here in **Benched V**, I'll tell you about all the causes of vaginitis that are unrelated to the non-sexually transmitted ailments in **Cranky V.**)

Vaginitis, the medical term to describe an inflamed vagina, incorporates what I like to term as The Big 3 Types: **Candidiasis** (yeast), **Bacterial Vaginosis**, and **Vulvovaginal Atrophy**. There is a lot of overlap in the symptoms of each of these conditions, so determination of the culprit can be confusing, which is why I prefer my patients to come into the office for a vaginal culture and pelvic exam to make certain of the correct diagnosis. If you're using *Grandma Sadie's yogurt remedy* to treat what may actually be a bacterial infection instead of a yeast infection, you may be waiting a very long time before you experience relief!

Typical symptoms of vaginitis include vulvar itching, burning, redness, and swelling, which may or may not be accompanied by vaginal discharge. If discharge is apparent, it can be white, yellow, or grey, thin, thick, or lumpy. To make diagnosis more confusing, sometimes there is a vaginal odor and sometimes there isn't!

The Most Popular Culprit: Candidaisis (Yeast)

By far the most popular and common type of vaginitis is **yeast** (more commonly referred to as a yeast infection). Normally, the bacteria of the vagina prevent yeast from overgrowing, but when their efforts fail, the delicate balance of the vagina is disrupted and *voila!* Yeast.

The main symptoms of candidiasis are itching, thick white vaginal discharge, and a red and swollen vulva, while odor is not a common symptom. A simple vaginal culture can identify this infection. Treatment can then include over-the-counter vaginal Monistat or prescription oral fluconazole (Diflucan). The problem is that women typically self-diagnose their symptoms as yeast, when oftentimes the cause is **bacterial vaginosis (BV)**, requiring a completely different treatment.

Laura, 31, loves her job, her life, and Frank, her steady boyfriend of four years. She was already on her back, feet in the stirrups when I walked into the exam room for a last minute office visit. Vibrant, outspoken and never one to mince words, she raised her head and blurted out, "Can you smell that shit! I smell like I've been fishing all day off Santa Monica Pier! Frank went down on me and was like, there's something wrong with your cooch!" I had to admit that I detected the smell the minute I walked into the room. It was almost like a thick cloud over her body. Assuming she had a yeast infection she'd tried one course of Monistat and one course of Diflucan (after a frenzied call to my nurse, Dani, for a prescription) to no avail.

Bacterial Vaginosis (File Under: That Really Fishy Smell)

Imagine the normally occurring bacteria of the vagina existing peacefully when suddenly some outside factor rushes in and disrupts their gentle balance. What you have is vaginal chaos, or, more to the point, **BV**. Primary symptoms of bacterial infection are a strong, fishy odor and thin gray or green vaginal discharge. Itching tends not to be a symptom of BV, but sometimes yeast will co-pilot this type of infection.

Standard treatment includes vaginal or oral antibiotics such as Metronidazole and Clindamycin. As was the case with Laura, women often self-diagnose a yeast infection and believe they can manage with an over-the-counter remedy.

When that doesn't work, they're in my office a month later for what should have been their first line of defense, a vaginal culture, which would have determined BV. **VVL**

Sexually Transmitted Infections (STIs)

The cast of characters for this one is long and, unfortunately, diverse. It includes:

* Human Papilloma Virus (HPV)
* Chlamydia
* Gonorrhea
* Syphilis
* Herpes (HSV)
* Trichomoniasis
* Crabs/Pubic Lice
* Scabies
* HIV/AIDS
* Mycoplasma

Who Is At Risk?

STIs do not discriminate. They are spread from partner to partner by direct contact, similar to how a common cold is transmitted. At risk are those who have unprotected sex, multiple sex partners, a history of STI's, and those who are prone to alcohol or drug abuse, which affect *judgment*—a large deciding factor in contracting a sexually transmitted disease.

The Facts About STI

Recently it has been reported that twenty-five percent of sexually active teens and young adults 15–24 acquire almost *half* of all new sexually transmitted infections. Because of screening programs that tend to focus more on females, the rate of STIs looks to be higher in women than men. Adolescents who use alcohol or drugs are more likely to have unplanned and unprotected sex, which put them at a higher risk for contracting STIs, and half of them surveyed said that the main reason their peers don't use contraception is because of alcohol and drug use.

Most common amongst the STIs are Human Papillomavirus (HPV), Chlamydia, Gonorrhea, Herpes, HIV, Hepatitis B, and Syphilis, with women 20–24 having the greatest incidence of HPV. Women 14–19 were found to have a twenty-four percent prevalence of HPV.

There is good news on this front, though. Enter the **HPV vaccine**, which has been helpful in reducing the incidence of HPV infections by more than ninety percent. If only people weren't so afraid of this life-saving vaccine! You'll see what I mean in the next story!

HIV, Vaccinations, and the "Wisdom" of Justin Timberlake

Jennifer, a well-read, well-meaning, vegan yoga practitioner and teacher, has avoided "Western medicine" for most of her adult life. At fifty-three, she is also the mother of twin fourteen-year-old girls Samantha and Monica. Jennifer's Sikh doctor of twenty years had taken care of most of her and her twins' medical issues, but this particular day Jennifer was in my office with her girls to discuss the vaccine for the human papilloma virus (HPV), which she'd been reading so much about. "I read that it caused seizures in kids," she told me. "Plus Jenny McCarthy and now Justin Timberlake are recommending that kids avoid vaccines if possible." This was not the first (or second or third) time I'd heard this mantra regarding the Gardassil vaccine for **the most common sexually transmitted infection, HPV**. I explained to Jennifer that HPV is so common that almost every sexually active woman and man carry at least one type of HPV without even knowing it! Women with certain types of HPV are more likely to have Pap smear abnormalities and are at a greater risk for cervical cancer. More than seventy-nine million people currently have HPV, with fourteen million more contracting the virus each year. Jennifer's eyes remained wide, like a deer in headlights, as I ticked off the **facts** about HPV. Ironically, Samantha and Monica finally let me know that they were the ones who went to their mother arguing the importance of the vaccination (which is why they were all in my office). It was mom who had to be brought up to speed, not the teens! Jennifer was also relieved to learn that the information she'd heard about contracting HPV from toilet seats was also, decidedly, *mis*information.

HPV: The One Everyone is Talking About

Human papillomavirus (HPV) is the most common sexually transmitted infection, affecting ninety percent of women and eighty percent of men, causing, among other things, genital warts, cervical, and oral cancers. HPV is epidemic! Your risk of exposure is directly related to the number of sexual partners you have had. The more partners you or your partner have had, the greater your risk of exposure to HPV. Primarily associated with vaginal, cervical, vulvar, penile and anal warts, HPV is also responsible for cervical pre-cancer and malignant cancers in women. Less common—but generating a lot of news and conversation—is a link between HPV and head, neck, throat, mouth, and anal cancers, for which men are equally at risk (in addition to penile cancer). In fact, HPV accounts for a higher incidence of anal carcinoma in those engaging in anal sex, resulting in a higher prevalence in gay men. Anal Pap smears are controversial in their accuracy, but they are indeed an option for men and women engaging in anal intercourse with a history of HPV exposure.

Out of the *more than 100 different types of HPV* (some of which do not cause health problems), there are forty or so types that can affect the vagina, penile, and anal areas, often resulting in pre-cancer changes. Because HPV is contracted through skin-to-skin contact, typically during sex, it's best to avoid sexual partners with genital warts or a known history of HPV. The problem with that advice is that most people are unaware that they carry HPV, especially men. Unfortunately, men do not have an equivalent to the Pap smear, which allows detection of HPV. Unless men have warts or a history of warts, they have no way of detecting this epidemic virus. Even a condom does not provide complete protection against HPV since the virus may live at the base of the penis or in other exposed areas, thereby allowing it to pass to the woman during sexual intercourse. Transmission of the virus can happen during vaginal or anal sex, oral sex, or hand-to-genital contact. Straight and same-sex couples are at equally high risk of HPV. Contrary to the misinformation out there, one cannot contract HPV by sharing a towel with a roommate or sitting on a toilet seat.

What's necessary in avoiding this disease is an open and honest conversation with your partner *prior to sex* about each other's sexually transmitted infection history.

Exposure to HPV

HPV is most commonly detected on a Pap smear screening during a routine gynecologic exam, since the Pap allows detection of abnormal or precancerous cells on the cervix. Unlike the herpes simplex virus, where symptoms of transmission are noticeable within days or weeks, it may take weeks or years after that first exposure to HPV for a Pap smear to turn up abnormal. Until then, most women don't have any other symptoms of HPV, and they may have been exposed to many different types of HPV through any number of different partners. It's only when the doctor's office calls to say, "We found the HPV virus on you Pap smear," that a woman is first alerted!

The only real recognizable symptom of HPV is the presence of **genital warts**, which look like small, skin-colored or pink growths on the labia, vagina, anus, or penis. They're often described as looking like small cauliflowers and may appear singularly or in clusters. Once they are diagnosed through inspection or biopsy, they can be treated by excision or through medication such as Podophyllin or Trichloroacetic acid. The latter is typically repeated weekly for four to six weeks until the warts disappear. Unfortunately, the treatment of HPV warts rarely produces permanent results.

Do Not Be Afraid of the Life-Saving HPV Vaccine!

As I told Jennifer, the HPV vaccine has a very safe track record. Most important, latest studies show that within the six years since HPV vaccines have been introduced there has been a huge decrease in young women and teen girls contracting the highest-risk types of HPV. In young women twenty to twenty-four, there has been a thirty-four percent decrease, and in teens, fourteen to nineteen, a sixty-four percent decrease! **Gardasil 9**, the most recent HPV vaccine, can prevent 90% of the HPV high-risk types—6, 11, 16, 18, 31, 33, 45, 52 and 58. The rate of HPV-linked cancers, cervical for women and oral cancer for men, are on the rise and can be prevented by the HPV vaccine.

Most side effects of the vaccine are mild, such as pain, redness, and soreness in the arm where the shot was given. Other mild side effects may include fainting, dizziness, fever, headache, nausea, and muscle or joint pain. Some people have fainting spells and jerking movement after receiving the injection but this can happen with any type of medication given with a needle. And with any vaccination a rare anaphylactic allergic reaction can occur. In my humble opinion, these minor side effects are a small price to pay for such a large health advantage.

As the Center of Disease Control (CDC) puts it, "Full vaccination coverage of the U.S. population could prevent future HPV-attributable cancers."

The Twins: Chlamydia and Gonorrhea

We rarely hear about Chlamydia and Gonorrhea since HPV was co-opted by the media, but there are an estimated 2.8 million new infections of both each year. Young women ages 15–24 have the highest rate of these sexually transmitted diseases. But what's interesting is that both of these bacterial strains affect women more than men. Unfair, yes, I know. And symptoms of Chlamydia and Gonorrhea are not always obvious as often there's no apparent vaginal discharge or itching or odor. In fact, the majority of cases I diagnose each year are in women who have absolutely no idea they even have a vaginal infection, though some women may experience yellow discharge, vaginal bleeding in between periods, pain or infrequency of peeing, rectal bleeding, discharge, or pain.

Since these particular STIs may go undiagnosed for a long time—days, weeks, and even months—the bacteria from both has time to travel from the vagina to the cervix, into the uterus, and to the fallopian tubes and ovaries, causing **Pelvic Inflammatory Disease (PID)**. This disease affects fertility by causing irreversible scarring of the fallopian tubes (the delicate pipes that transmit the egg to be fertilized by sperm) and damage to the ovaries. One terrible PID infection can cause permanent infertility and increase the risk of tubal (ectopic) pregnancies. For this reason, it's recommended that women twenty-five and younger be screened yearly and after a change in sexual partners for Chlamydia and Gonorrhea.

If an early diagnosis of Chlamydia or Gonorrhea is made, antibiotics are the way to an easy, successful treatment both for you and *your partner*. Getting re-cultured is a must in order to ensure the complete disappearance of these fertility-disrupting bugs. Left untreated, this is the gift that keeps on giving!

Syphilis

Another bacteria spread through sexual contact is Syphilis—perhaps the most popular sexually transmitted disease of modern melodrama and theatre, probably because it ravaged much of sixteenth and seventeenth century Europe! Unlike Chlamydia and Gonorrhea, Syphilis is transmitted through a skin sore or painless chancre (dull, hard lesion or skin ulcer) on the vulva, vagina, anus, or penis on an infected person.

Benched V

The bacteria go through three different stages, progressively worsening. A painless genital chancre will eventually give way to a rash on the soles of the feet and palms of the hands, followed by flu-like symptoms and, possibly, flat warts on the vulva. The last stage of the disease comes after the rash and other symptoms disappear, when the bacteria goes dormant in the body, ultimately manifesting itself in heart or neurologic problems, blindness, paralysis, tumors, brain damage, or death.

So what's the good news after hearing these grim prospects? Syphilis can be diagnosed during a physical exam or from a blood test. Once the diagnosis is made, antibiotics are given to avoid any catastrophic medical problems (no such luck in the jolly seventeenth Century). Notifying all sexual partners is crucial after such a diagnosis.

Alexandria (Alex) has been my patient since she was sixteen. A straight A+ student throughout high school, she was determined to go to UCLA, with a scholarship, which she handily achieved—although, through-the-roof SAT scores, a volunteering stint in an African orphanage, and authoring a children's book may also had something to do with that accomplishment. At twenty-six, Alex was graduating with her master's in public health with a sense of determination that equaled her good humor. Yes, you know what's coming. STI's can happen to anyone. Anyone. Alex had called the office in between her regular visits. She'd been crying when she got on the phone with my nurse, Dani. When I spoke to her she was "really fucking pissed off" that her boyfriend had gone down on her with a cold sore in his mouth, something she hadn't initially noticed. She was too shocked to believe what was happening, but when she described a fever and flu-like symptoms four days after that fateful not-so-romantic encounter, and "a thousand blisters" on her vagina preventing her from leaving the house or peeing without horrible pain, I knew enough. She even sent me a vagina selfie, which confirmed my suspicion that she had indeed contracted genital herpes. Although necessary, the pelvic exam and viral culture seemed almost an afterthought. **VVL**

Herpes Simplex Virus (HSV)

The herpes simplex virus affects an estimated forty-five million women and men in the U.S. alone. Unfortunately, knowing how common an STI it is certainly didn't make Alex feel any better. As informed as she was, she'd never thought to ask whether her boyfriend (now "former") had any cold or canker sores in his mouth before their sexual encounter.

There are two strains of herpes, Type 1 and Type 2 (HSV-1 and HSV-2). Herpes Type 1 is oral herpes that appears as a cold sore (also known as a fever blister) on the lips, nose or face, or as a canker sore in the mouth or on the tongue. It begins as a blister, which eventually breaks open and starts to ooze. After a week or so, the ulcer-like sore crusts over, leaving a scab, which will then take a while to heal completely. During most of this time the sore is considered *active,* which means that the virus may be passed on to *you* or *your partner.*

If you've been exposed to herpes Type I it may take up to twenty days for the sores to even show up. You may notice a tingling or itching sensation in the area where the sore will develop. Once the virus in in your system, stress, fever, colds, illness, sunburns and even your period can trigger an outbreak.

Type 2 herpes *originates* in the genital area and can be passed to one's partner through genital-to-genital contact. If you have HSV-1 (a cold sore on your lip) and you perform oral sex on your partner, you can pass Type 1 to the genital area. Oral herpes is readily transmitted to the genitals during oral sex!

As of this writing, there are no approved vaccines to prevent herpes, but medications such as Valtrex and Acyclovir can be used to prevent an outbreak, or can be utilized at the very onset of one to curtail the severity of symptoms.

Trichomoniasis (Trich)

Pronounced: *Trick*. It may feel like one, but it certainly isn't funny. Trichomoniasis is actually a very common (and very curable) STI transmitted by a microscopic parasite through sexual contact. Symptoms may include yellow-gray or green vaginal discharge along with the characteristic fishy odor associated with the infection. Vaginal burning, redness, irritation and swelling may also be present. Treatment for Trich is with a one-time oral dose of the prescription antibiotic metronidazole (Flagyl). You cannot drink alcohol when taking this drug, as it may cause severe nausea and vomiting, but know that you will be cured. Just remember that your sexual partner must also be treated for the infection since it is sexually transmitted.

Advice on How to Avoid Being Benched

* Choose your partners carefully (RULE 1!)
* Always have your partner wear a condom
* Try to limit the number of sexual partners

* If you see any sores on your partner's genitals or mouth, AVOID contact with them (the sores, maybe not necessarily the partner)
* See your healthcare provider if you have any symptoms such as unusual vaginal discharge, itching, or pelvic pain
* Get yearly STI testing
* STI testing *in between partners* is vital
* Practice good communication with your partner *before* becoming intimate, which leads us to...

KISS and TELL (This One Warrants Its Own Heading)

It is so necessary to have that completely awkward conversation with a new partner if you have a Benched V—I would hope that your new partner (male or female) would have the decency to give you likewise information as well. Chances are your partner will have a newfound respect for your honesty (if not, it's a good thing to find that out early in the game!). Especially if you've been exposed in the past to HPV and/or Herpes, you must inform your partner of that fact since these are the two most easily sexually transmitted STIs.

I'd suggest having this conversation *before* you have a couple of drinks and *before* you've strewn your clothes around the room. Have it on a date or during dinner if you feel the relationship is heading towards sexual intimacy.

Honesty is the best policy, especially in the bedroom! Make it part of your *dating routine* to bring up the subject of STIs. As unromantic as it may seem, make it a priority even before *kissing*.

Your Priorities

Top of the list: *Healthy Living.*

For healthy living you need to take control of what you put in your mouth as well as what you put in your vagina. Speaking of which, **condoms** are the best way to help prevent sexually transmitted infections, pregnancy, HIV infections, and related diseases such as cervical cancer. Truly, most Benched Vs can be prevented with condom use. No, it's not one hundred percent protection, but if you're sexually active it *is* your best chance of preventing unwanted surprises. I implore you, make a pledge to have your new or old partner wear a condom at all times until you make the decision to be completely monogamous. Why take the chance of being thrown a curveball by your healthcare provider—a call informing you that, yes, you've won the STI lottery! *Congratulations, you've quite possibly affected your future fertility (not to mention health) and need a round of antibiotics ASAP!*

In hindsight (a wonderful thing, hindsight), I'm pretty sure the only reason I avoided STIs in my youth was because I was so overly cautious about having sex...with anyone. I was waiting for that special person to come along, unsure of whether it would be a man or a woman. I lost my virginity to the man I married (I didn't even think to ask him to wear a condom), and then I figured since I had sex with him I ought to really try to make the relationship work despite my own uncertainties about our future together. I was a naïve, confused, and impulsive young woman, and I was going through my own sexual identity crisis. I only wish that I'd had a doctor who asked me a few tough questions about my own sexual health and identity or one who, at least, advised me on safe sex.

It was assumed that I knew my body, my mind, and my vagina. And never, despite the signs (obvious now, in that damned hindsight) did anyone question my sexual preference.

I say to you, *out of experience,* find a healthcare provider who can be your sexual health "wing-man"—someone who will help you negotiate your sexual well-being. Ask yourself if you truly know the definition of "safe sex." If it doesn't come to mind as quickly as your bankcard password, then you are *not* ready to be sexually intimate with anyone. Safe sex means condom use during vaginal or anal intercourse and oral sex (during which dental dams are used to protect the throat from HPV). And if there isn't a dental dam in grabbing distance, plastic wrap or a cut condom will do the trick. Creativity counts, ladies.

Don't be sidelined. A **Benched V** is often *preventable.* Pay attention to your vagina and your overall lifestyle. Don't be afraid to ask questions. You and your **V** will win out in the long run.

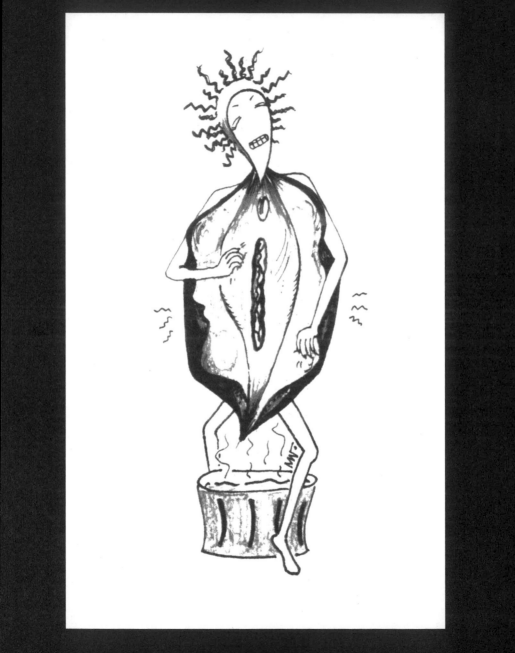

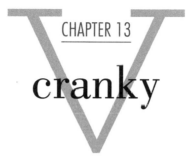

CHAPTER 13

cranky

66 I was in my late twenties when I entered motherhood—a time when most of my friends weren't even *thinking* of kids—so I didn't have any girlfriends with good advice on the subject. My husband and I took the obligatory birth class, which provided us with instructions on which hospital door to enter through (the front one, not the emergency entrance), what to pack in my overnight bag, and how to install an infant car seat—I think I daydreamed my way through the actual baby birthing part of the class. Our plan? Well, it was to have our baby—little did we know he had a plan of his own.

In my ninth month of pregnancy my baby wedged his foot between my ribs and managed to crack my rib cage, which meant that lying prone was out of the question, so from then on I had to sleep sitting straight up. I was probably a little delirious when, a week past my due date, I convinced Dr. Sherry Ross to induce me. After four epidurals, my boy came tearing out, literally—his name was supposed to be Hudson, but, roughed up as he was, with only one eye open, my husband suggested he seemed more like a "Jack." Believe me, the pushing part of giving birth was a piece of cake compared to the recovery, which took almost a year. From the moment I felt that memorable stitch pop, a day or so after Jack's grand entrance into the world, I had to deal with a very cranky V. I will spare you the gory details of my recovery, other than to say that during it I became pregnant with my second child, Ava!

Ava was our "surprise" baby—a very happy surprise, but a surprise nonetheless. We hadn't planned on getting pregnant again so soon after Jack, and since the first time was so traumatic, and I hadn't fully healed "down there," I vowed I'd have a C-section. Even though all was right with my equipment by the time my due date arrived, the memories of Jack's birth were vivid enough for me to stay the C-section course.

Until I was pregnant I basically avoided going to the doctor. I was never the alarmist type. My attitude was such that if I wasn't bleeding profusely from a head wound, whatever ailment I had would eventually go away. I figured, why bother making an unnecessary trip to *the doctor*?

Since my pregnancies, my relationship with Dr. Sherry Ross has made me a doctor appointment convert. I actually look forward to my yearly visits—which are more like pilgrimages because I live on the opposite side of town and have to navigate hours of horrendous Los Angeles traffic. What's ironic is that reading this chapter of Dr. Sherry Ross' book made me realize that it doesn't make sense not to check in with a doctor when something is troubling. I mean, come on—and I say this to myself as well—there's no need to tough it out on your own when dealing with something as important as your V and your health in general.

Cranky V

My daughter, Ava, is almost 10, which means she's only a few years away from seeing Dr. Sherry Ross for her own exams. Even though the idea of that is beyond crazy to me right now—it makes me feel super old—I feel super assured that she will be in the best hands possible. I want her to never hesitate to check in with her doctor—our doctor—about any concerns she may have about her own body. So, if you're reading this, don't you hesitate either. 99

—Amy Acker Actress

At thirty-seven, Sonia is a single woman and one of the top advertising execs for Google. Her job requires more travel days a year than she'd prefer, but like she says, "Hell, I'm not complaining." Well, that's not necessarily true, because as much as I love Sonia, she is a casebook hypochondriac. In the few years that Sonia's been my patient I've had to talk her off a ledge when she's called with a migraine, convinced of a brain tumor. A sudden pain in her breast? Cancer. Stomach? Cancer. The truth is that Sonia is a lean, healthy woman with an enviable physique. However, there was one thing that Sonia was not imagining. Often I'd get a call from her while she was on layover somewhere across the country, and she'd be pissed! "My va-jay-jay is like a ball of fire!" She'd ask me to call something in to the pharmacy nearest her hotel. Before starting to see me, she'd been around town to several gynecologists with what she described as "the itchiest crotch in Los Angeles." She told me, "No one can tell me why! I've had every test there is!" Last time she called me she said, "I had to leave an office meeting the other day to go scratch myself in the bathroom. I scratched so hard that I started to bleed. What the hell is going on down there?" Again, the vaginal cultures proved negative.

Cease and desist that urge to itch! Please don't automatically assume you have a yeast infection as you run with your Cranky V to the local CVS for some over the counter Monistat or Vagisil. You create an uphill battle by playing doctor and missing a true diagnosis—treatment is delayed and your vagina may become so angry and painful that your Cranky V is all you can think of. Over the years the most painful vaginas I've treated are those suffering from what is called the "itch-scratch" cycle (which we will go into in this chapter). If you are suffering from an itchy crotch for more than a week, promise me you'll GO SEE YOUR HEALTHCARE PROVIDER so that you may start to...

...Itch No More

Okay, your doctor has ruled out a yeast or bacterial infection, so what the heck is making your vagina itch so? Once you've gotten the clear, literally, on your vaginal culture, it's time to look for another cause of what is known as the "itch-scratch" cycle, a most irritating condition if there ever was one. There may not be an actual source, but there are environmental issues that worsen the discomfort and symptoms of the cycle.

Fragrant body and laundry soaps, sanitary pads, and stress are some of the main culprits. Unfortunately, by the time you show up in your health provider's office with this condition the itching is likely to the point of "severe and intractable." The only remedy seems to be to scratch, which only serves to worsen the itch! After cultures have ruled out infection, it becomes time to break the "itch-scratch" cycle with aggressive treatment. Daily gentle steroid cream, moisturizing baths, and other medicated balms can restore the health and integrity of the vaginal tissue, thus breaking the cycle and bringing relief to the rescue.

Sonia's case required just a little detective work. I discovered that she always wore a thin mini-pad because of a light vaginal discharge, especially during her business trips. Her mother had told her to wear the pad so that her panties wouldn't get stained—even at thirty-seven we're still listening to our mothers, which can be good and not so good. Seems that the mini-pads were the culprit. Sonia's business trips were great for frequent flyer miles but a nightmare for her sensitive V. **VVL**

Have a Vagina? Then You've Probably Experienced "the Itch."

It's a common occurrence, that disruptive and embarrassing thing known as the "itch-scratch" cycle, a condition of the vulva unrelated to a typical yeast or bacterial infection. Seventy percent of women have vaginal itching at one time or another, but the oft-ignored "itch-scratch" cycle affects twenty-five percent of women. The truth is that anywhere on our bodies where there is skin, nerve fibers, hair/hair follicles, and sweat glands there is a potential for itching. Environmental factors that create heat, sweating, rubbing, frictions, and other forms of mild trauma can contribute to that annoying V-itch. So, yes, basically living can be the cause.

As soon as that itch-scratch becomes disruptive and noticeable throughout the day or night it is time to see your healthcare provider. Vulvar itching may be caused by normal environmental conditions such as the ones mentioned, or it can be the result of an underlying organic *medical* condition.

Typical medical organic conditions that may cause vulvar itching include:

* Yeast and bacterial infections
* Lichen Simplex Chronicus
* Psoriasis
* Contact dermatitis
* Latex allergy
* HPV-warts
* Vulvar Intraepithelial dysplasia
* Vulvar Atrophy related to Menopause

Before making a diagnosis of "scratch-itch" cycle, organic conditions, such as those mentioned, need to be ruled out. **VVL**

Chronic Scratch-Itch Cycle

Lichen Simplex Chronicus (LSC) is the medical condition most commonly known as the itch-scratch cycle. It's a condition that can be very confusing. The first step for a healthcare provider in making this diagnosis is to take a thorough history from the patient. Likely in this history a patient has been itching for weeks or months. When she finally seeks medical evaluation, the itching is likely severe and unmanageable— the only thing that feels good is to scratch! Scratching often occurs on a subconscious level during the day and night, while sleeping, and can result in abrasions and tears if left untreated. Often under-recognized by the clinician but largely connected to this condition are psychological factors such as anxiety and depression, although it is the skin irritants that often start the cycle.

Something as simple as wearing tight underwear or jeans can start the itch that never seems to abate. With chronic itching comes thickening and drying of the skin, which promotes the itch-scratch cycle, which, in turn, lead to visible changes on the hood of the clitoris, the lips of the vagina and the area around the anus. Changes may also include lightening or darkening of the vulvar skin, grayish white and thicker skin, fissures, and hair loss. Heat, stress, mini-pads, lubricants, fragrant soaps and laundry products, and menses exacerbate the symptoms. **VVL**

Once it's determined by a healthcare provider that you do not have a yeast or bacterial infection or some other medical condition and an itch-scratch cycle has been diagnosed, there are ways to treat this chronic condition.

Banishing the Itch and Breaking the Cycle

First in the line of battle is the use of a gentle **steroid cream** that will not thin the skin of the vagina (and worsen the symptoms). At the same time, it's important to use a natural moisturizer to hydrate the sensitive skin of the vulva. I recommend a daily twenty-minute bath with Aveeno bath powder, which helps to moisturize and hydrate the vulva's irritated, dry skin. A handful of extra virgin coconut oil in the bath also works well in hydrating skin tissue. I suggest these nightly baths for two to three weeks, along with a gentle daily steroid cream. Alternately, I've found great success with a compounded medicated cream that includes hydrocortisone 2%, Estriol .05%, and lidocaine 5% in an Aquaphor base for two weeks.

Once the scratch-itch cycle has been interrupted with the bath/cream therapy, I would suggest continuing the Aveeno bath 2–3 times a week, with the steroid cream as needed. Calmoseptine cream is also helpful in treating the itch.

More aggressive therapy may include—aside from daily baths and hydrating cream—*moderately strong* topical steroids, daily anti-itch oral medication such as Doxepin, short-term systemic steroids, and/or antidepressants and serotonin inhibitors such as Amitriptyline.

Whatever the treatment, be mindful in minimizing or avoiding the environmental factors that may aggravate symptoms. If a psychological component such as anxiety or depression is the underlying cause, appropriate therapy will be necessary to prevent a recurrence. Still not sure what factors may be a problem?

Common Vulvar Irritants You May or May Not Realize Are Problematic

* Fragrant soaps, bubble bath liquids, bath salts
* Detergents, fabric softeners, and dryer sheets
* Sanitary wipes and pads
* Warming gels and scented lubricants
* Nylon underwear or wet bathing suits
* Post-workout sweaty gym clothes
* Rubber products such as diaphragms and condoms
* Saliva or semen (I kid you not)
* Spermicides such as foams, creams, and jellies
* Feminine hygiene sprays, tampons, or deodorant pads
* Creams or ointments applied to the vulva

A useful tip for all is: best to wear cotton or microfiber underwear during the day. At night, give your vulva a chance to *breathe* and chuck the panties altogether.

Keep the Balance—Don't Mess with Your V's pH

Suzy and Larry were sixteen years married and monogamous. At forty-eight, Suzy was a long-term social worker in the Los Angeles community of Watts with the kind of dedication that made Suzy's office wish for forty more like her. Unfortunately for Suzy, it was her third visit to my office for the same foul-smelling green discharge that had plagued her previously. This time she revealed something she hadn't before: "I've been douching to get rid of the awful smell—along with taking the prescription for Metrogel—but it keeps coming back! What else can I do for this nasty thing?"

Bacterial vaginosis (BV) is a common condition that can drive a patient crazy, as it's difficult to treat. But first, *stop douching,* is what I told Suzy (for more of why douching is never the answer, please take a peek at Chapter 1 on the **Healthy V**). The normally acidic vagina usually keeps bacterial vaginosis away; however, when the pH balance is disrupted, BV may present itself with symptoms that include a thin, grayish-white discharge and an intense, foul-smelling odor. During intercourse, the mixture of ejaculate and the BV bacteria can create the classic "fishy" smell. Once a vaginal culture confirms the diagnosis, treatment with the oral antibiotics metronidazole (generic for Metrogel) or clindamycin would be effective. **VVL**

Since Suzy had already taken Metrogel, her first recommended treatment, it was time to offer an alternative. Half of all women who have been treated for BV will have a recurrence within the first year. Chronic sufferers, fear not. If Metrogel does not provide relief, I would suggest clindamycin cream, applied vaginally at bedtime for seven days.

It can be difficult to identify the cause of BV, but risk factors include African American ethnicity, sexual intercourse, and douching. BV is commonly seen with yeast infections.

Following treatment, it's always best to get re-cultured to make certain the treatment was a success. You may also want to use vaginal boric acid capsules, which can be made by a compounding pharmacy. They're a safe and effective means of maintaining a healthy pH balance.

Chronic Candidiasis

Yeast. We rarely want to hear about it unless it has to do with bread. But candidiasis—more commonly known as **yeast infections**—is the most common cause of vaginitis in women. However, *chronic yeast infection* does *not* refer to the vaginal itching and cottage cheese-like discharge that is easily vanquished with an over-the-counter treatment of Monistat or prescription antifungal such as Diflucan (to which certain strains of candida are resistant).

Chronic yeast refers to *four or more* symptomatic cases of *candida vulvovaginitis* (vaginal yeast infection) in a 12-month period. Symptoms include chronic vaginal pain along with intense itching and thick discharge. Those who may be prone to chronic yeast include women who have frequent sex (like this should ever be a problem?), women with new partners, and those who have recently taken or tend to take antibiotics. A vaginal culture can and should confirm the diagnosis of chronic yeast. **VVL**

Treatment for recurrent infections include:

* Oral fluconazole
* Boric acid capsules

Cranky V

* Flucystosine, another vaginal medication made by a compounding pharmacy

Again, as with treatment for any vaginal condition, it's best to get re-cultured to insure that the treatment was, indeed, successful.

Ladies, it is not normal to have to leave an event or find a private corner of a room to scratch your vagina as though you're suffering from having gone dancing naked through a field of thigh-high Poison Ivy. There are so many possible causes for a Cranky V, and most often only a healthcare provider can solve the mystery of your interminable itch. Don't let your vagina remain chronically cranky. Give it the little bit of patience and TLC it obviously craves.

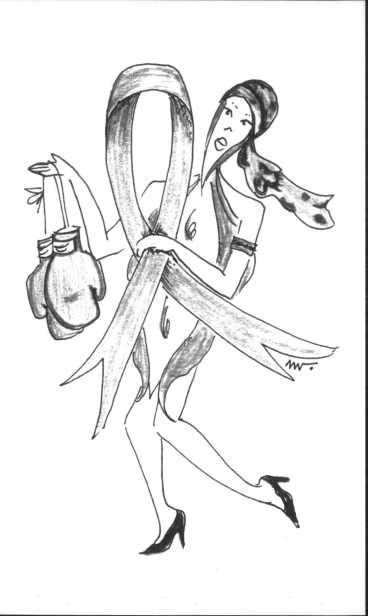

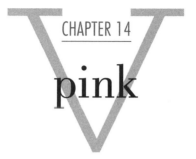

CHAPTER 14

pink

66 When your doctor (in my case, Dr. Sherry Ross) calls to tell you about the results of your recent mammogram and the first thing she says is "Where are you right now?" you pretty much know it's not going to be good news. I got that call when I was on my way to buy a new refrigerator. So there, in the parking lot of Home Depot, while I sat in my car staring blankly at the outdoor display of Bar-B-Que grills, I got the not so good news. And then, in the first of what would be many "screw you, cancer" moves, I went inside and bought myself a damned refrigerator. Not even cancer would force me to make two trips to Home Depot.

The preliminary reports came in on a Friday morning, and I was not going to get any specific information about my cancer until Monday afternoon. You learn a lot about yourself when you have three days to live in the dark unknown of a "C" word diagnosis.

She·ology

I learned that I don't like to feel sorry for myself. I learned I wouldn't be able to bear thirty people calling me daily to ask how I am. I learned why doctors don't recommend looking up your ailments on the Internet. I learned that a twenty-year-old episode of *Oprah*, featuring Erin Kramp—a woman dying of breast cancer who left a legacy of videos to her husband and daughter for all the major events she would miss—was indelibly etched into my brain. I thought of the videos I would leave for my son, Milo. I also learned that in spite of my fear I will never miss a party—and I had two fabulous parties to go to that weekend.

For two weeks I didn't tell anyone I had cancer. I had so much to learn about my particular cancer that I didn't want to split my energy between researching doctors, surgeons, and treatments and having to explain my story over and over again. Once I had a better understanding of my options I wrote this letter to my girlfriends, two days before my 55th birthday—Hell, if I'm being honest about cancer I might as well be honest about my age.

Dear Ones,

I cannot wait to see you all on Sunday for my birthday dinner.

I just wanted to let you know what was going on with me. I'm sorry I'm doing it through an email, but to be perfectly honest, I'm just too exhausted to explain this to each of you individually. Please do not forward this email to anyone. Of course you can talk amongst yourselves. It's no fun if you can't.

About a week and a half ago I was diagnosed with breast cancer. Big Bummer.

I had a routine mammogram and they noticed a curious spot in my left breast. I had an MRI, then a biopsy and it was determined I have invasive ductal carcinoma, which sounds way worse than it is. I only have stage 2A cancer and it's totally curable.

Pink V

I will have a substantial lumpectomy mid-March and they will have to do a bit of a reconstruction/reduction to make them even sized. So I will get some gorgeous breasts out of it. (Yay, Silver Lining!) They will also take out a few lymph nodes during the surgery and depending on the results, the doctor will determine if I will need chemo or radiation.

I spent all last week meeting three separate teams of cancer surgeons, plastic surgeons, radiology oncologists, medical oncologists, and getting my pre-op work done. I have picked a great team and I know I am in excellent hands.

I am very optimistic. It's not going to be fun, except for the new boobs part, but I caught it early enough that my prognosis is excellent. One in eight women get breast cancer, so I'm taking one for the team. You can thank me in jewelry.

Feel free to call, text, email, send chocolate. I don't really have any more info than what I've just told you, though I will say this: I am truly humbled by the collective strength and courage of my gender. From the few women I've talked to about their experience with breast cancer, to the all-female-team of surgeons I have put in place, to the testimonials I've read, to the handful of women who have known what I've gone through this past week, I have never felt more connected to this mighty sisterhood. Just writing this email and knowing it will land in your inboxes and that your blessings, wishes, and love will come my way gives me strength.

I love you and I can't wait to see you on Sunday.
xoxoxoxox Camryn 🙶

—Camryn Manheim Actress

She-ology

At thirty-four, Tabitha was diagnosed with leukemia a month before her marriage to Billy, her longtime boyfriend. Instead of a honeymoon on the beaches of Bora Bora working on the perfect tan, she was in the Angeles Clinic receiving her second cycle of chemotherapy. By her last round of chemo, she'd become accustomed to wrapping her bald head in beautiful, bright, floral scarves, and she'd captured the hearts of her oncology nurses with her easy, sweet smile and lack of complaints. When we were alone, though, she couldn't hold back the tears. I squeezed her hand and she said in a whisper, "Will I ever be able to use my vagina for sex again? Since the diagnosis we've only had sex twice. It's impossible, sex. There isn't enough KY jelly in the world to help us. It's so painful!"

For more than twenty years the pink ribbon has been used to raise awareness and funding for breast cancer, but for me, the ubiquity of the symbol is a reminder of cancer in any form—breast, colon, leukemia, lymphoma, melanoma, cervical, thyroid, uterine, etc.—as well as a reminder of how much it sucks. We all know that the scourge of cancer reaches across demographics, but what you may not be aware of is the fact that cancer is the leading cause of disease death in adolescents and young adults ages 15–39.

As has been pointed out to me time and time again, sex can be hard enough to talk about even with your girlfriends on a second round of happy hour Lemon Drops, so to talk about it with your doctor may be daunting, at best. Toss in sexual dysfunction as a side effect of cancer and the conversation can seem downright inconceivable. Between the embarrassment of the topic and the rushed nature of obligatory exams, there doesn't seem to be an opportune time to properly discuss something this important and sensitive.

One in three women will be diagnosed with cancer during their lifetime, of which sixty-four percent will experience the disease in a way that directly affects sexual organs. It's no wonder that sexual dysfunction is so common among cancer survivors. A survey by the Lance Armstrong Foundation found that forty-three percent of women had problems with sexual function following cancer treatment. Twenty-nine percent reported "a lot" of functional impairment. Sadly, of the entire group, only thirteen percent discussed their sexual dysfunction with their healthcare provider. This is definitely not an acceptable statistic. Communication is key in addressing the sexual problems resulting from cancer treatment which most commonly include:

* Loss of sexual desire.
* Failure to become sexually aroused.
* Vaginal dryness from premature menopause.
* Pain with sexual activity and intercourse.
* Problems with orgasms.
* Emotional changes created by poor body image and feelings of unattractiveness.
* Physical changes, including weight gain or loss, hair loss, swelling from lymphedema, skin sensitivities affecting the body's response to touch.
* Scars and ports, which create further body insecurities.

When these women were asked why they did not receive care for their post-cancer issues, just over half said that they'd simply learned to live with the problem. Thirty-seven percent were told that their issues were unavoidable side effects, twenty percent said they addressed the problems on their own, nineteen percent were told nothing could be done to help, and fourteen percent said they expected to get care sometime at a future date.

Even doctors who are open to *discussing* delicate sexual concerns agree that there is a real disconnect when it comes to a doctor's ability to start up a conversation about (gasp) vaginas and sex and dysfunction. One expert stated, "If you plan on waiting for your doctor to bring up the topic, it may be like waiting for hell to freeze over." Post cancer sexuality is still the elephant in the room!

Three Frightening Words

You have cancer. In the wake of these words, not only will your personal strength be tested, the strength and resilience of your relationship will be challenged in ways you could never have imagined. The newer a relationship, the more challenging such a diagnosis will be. With survival at the forefront of your thoughts, it's not surprising that your sexuality takes a back seat. The emotional toll is often as devastating as the physical one, as intimacy and sexual desire is overshadowed by that killjoy of all killjoys, **depression**. Depression is different from sadness—which you may also be experiencing. It's a serious mental health issue that robs you of hope and leaves you feeling lifeless and empty, which is why it is so important to open up to your partner about your feelings, to let them know how the cancer is affecting you both mentally and physically. A couples' therapist who specializes in cancer patients is also recommended, along with support groups that can help navigate the uncharted territory of a cancer diagnosis.

Of course, it's equally important to talk to your oncologist and your gynecologist about your concerns. They can help with your issues around sexual dysfunction, or at least provide avenues of support.

Tabitha...A Success Story

I'm happy to say that Tabitha did beat her cancer, but as a result of chemo she went into premature ovarian failure, which thrust her into early menopause at thirty-four. Fortunately, she had the child she'd always wanted—from a first marriage—and she and Billy knew early on that they didn't want more children, but her loss of sexual desire, her feelings of unattractiveness, and her excruciating vaginal dryness was preventing her from having sex with her husband of only four months. She was a basket case, worrying about losing her husband, "the man of her dreams." I knew it was her depression talking, exacerbated by her unfamiliar vagina! I had her buy vaginal dilators and I received approval from her oncologist for the prescription of vaginal estrogen three times weekly so that her vagina would be hydrated in preparation to resume some sexual activity. Tabitha used those dilators religiously. As she felt better, she even joked about the estrogen being like "watering her lady garden." After a couple months, she was able to resume sexual intercourse with Billy. With the dryness and pain treated, her sexual appetite returned, as did a healthy sexual relationship with her husband.

Cancer and the Under-Forty Set

Cancer patients between the ages of fifteen and thirty-nine tend to have different issues and concerns about their diagnosis than their older counterparts. The cancers most commonly afflicting women in this group are breast, ovarian, cervical, uterine and hematologic (such as Hodgkin's, Non-Hodgkin's, Leukemia). Some hospitals, like the University of Texas MD Anderson Cancer Center, have programs designed specifically to help deal with the age-specific problems of women younger than forty, whose most common issues include:

* They feel alone
* They've rarely met or even seen another patient their own age going through the same ordeal
* They've lost their independence and are relying on their parents again
* They're isolated from friends due to treatment
* As survivors, their friendships may have changed through the cancer treatment and they find themselves with an experience that few of their peers can understand or relate to

It's tragic for anyone to feel completely alone, but it's even more so when one feels hopeless and alone after a diagnosis of cancer. There are conscientious physicians and support groups out there to lead and buoy you through your cancer journey. Ask for help. Make your feelings known.

"Eight years ago, after testing positive for the breast cancer gene (BRCA), I was determined to change what seemed like a certain destiny to develop breast cancer. Having seen my mother battle breast cancer in her forties, and my mother-in-law succumb to the disease in her early fifties, I refused to accept the probable risk. I was inspired to test for the gene by one incredible woman's book, *Pretty is What Changes*. Even though I didn't personally know the author, Jessica Queller, she was like a sister in battle. Her story gave me the faith and courage to move forward, as she had, slashing and burning risk along the way. Jessica Queller was the first of many pioneers who guided me on my journey.

My next major inspiration on this journey was the incredible Dr. Sherry Ross. We had been through a lot together prior to my testing— my son's delivery with a surprise cleft lip and the birth of my twins seventeen months later, with one of the girls landing in intensive care for two weeks—so when Sherry called to say I had tested positively for the BRCA gene our conversation was surprisingly calm. I was ready for the news, and her confidence in our next steps gave me faith.

I underwent a double mastectomy and had my ovaries removed, but I don't know why I thought it would be less physically challenging than it actually was. With three small children and a full time job, I refused to imagine I would (or could) be out of commission for more than a few weeks—I told my bosses I'd be back at work in two! In reality, the surgery kicked my butt and I needed more than a month of recovery. The good news was that I was *mentally* prepared because I was so committed to living a long life for my husband and kids, and to doing everything humanly possible to ward off cancer. Seeing my mom's and my mother-in-law's battle with the disease, and having watched my dad's decade-long struggle with lung cancer made my path very clear.

Remarkably, in the subsequent years, my three sisters all tested positive for the gene. They are at various junctures in their individual journeys but they are all moving forward to reduce their risk. It's a rare occurrence for four sisters to claim the 50/50 odds cancer gene, but we have bonded as we've shared our experiences and encouraged our daughters (and sons) to be informed and to be aware of their own possible risks.

My now teenage daughters are already advocates for breast health, and they move forward with eyes wide open. I wish for a cure before my daughters have to make these major decisions, but for now, at least, I've armed them with the message that love, strength, support, and knowledge can get you through anything.

I'm so proud to be invited to be part of this incredible book. I know that *She-ology* and, especially, the Pink V chapter, will touch women who are at risk and walk readers calmly through it all—just as Dr. Sherry has done for me! 99

—Jennifer Nicholson-Salke President of Entertainment, NBC

Klara remembers her cancer diagnosis like it was yesterday. While showering she'd felt a penny-sized lump on her right breast, which led to a mammogram and subsequent biopsy, confirming Stage 3A breast cancer, BRCA1. (Stage 3 cancer means the breast cancer has extended to beyond the immediate region of the tumor and may have invaded nearby lymph nodes and muscles, but has not spread to distant organs. The difference of stages 3A, 3B, and 3C are determined by the size of the tumor and whether cancer has spread to the lymph nodes and surrounding tissue. BRCA1 is an inherited gene mutation that increases the risk not only of breast cancer, but ovarian as well.) At thirty-one, her formerly charismatic and optimistic self was crumbling. All she could say to me was, "Oh, my God, I want to be a mother! I want to get married! I want to live a long life!" Her surgeon performed a double mastectomy with implants and wanted to start chemo immediately following. Her team had recommended her ovaries be removed, since women who are BRCA1 positive have a greater risk for ovarian cancer. Wait—I know, she wanted kids! So her oncologist, breast surgeon, and I arranged with a fertility expert for Klara to freeze her eggs before her ovaries were obliterated by chemo.

The happy conclusion is that Klara is now six years cancer free. At her last yearly Pap smear, she brought her 18-month-old son Simon with her—thanks to one of her defrosted eggs, (unknown) donor sperm, and in vitro fertilization. Klara is also dating Teddy, her "soulmate," a man she met at her cancer support group. Teddy, in remission for Hodgkin's lymphoma, banked his sperm before his chemo treatments four years earlier. Klara and Teddy consider themselves the lucky ones—with a little luck and a lot of science, they will mix one of Klara's remaining eggs with Teddy's frozen sperm and have a child together.

You may have first heard of the BRCA gene from the highly publicized cancer diagnoses given to Christina Applegate and Angelina Jolie. Like Klara, both those women were younger than fifty when they tested positive for the gene. Both underwent double mastectomies and Angelina had her ovaries removed, which fortunately brought the issue of this genetic mutation right squarely into the public eye. Women facing the same diagnosis at such an early age have different life-changing decisions to make than other cancer victims. In particular, the women who are at a higher risk for this inherited form of breast and ovarian cancer have had one or more of the following:

* A breast cancer diagnosis before age fifty.
* Cancer in both breasts.
* Breast and ovarian cancer.
* Multiple breast cancers.

* Two or more primary types of BRCA1- or BRCA2-related cancers in a single family member.
* A family member with male breast cancer.
* Ashkenazi Jewish women with a single family member with breast or ovarian cancer before age fifty.

66 I will tell you the happy ending of this story first: Today my mother is a healthy, vibrant 75-year-old woman, but she was only forty when she was diagnosed with breast cancer. Fifteen years after treatment for the disease, she had an abnormal Pap smear. Although the abnormal cells had all the characteristics of ovarian cancer cells, doctors did not find cancer in her ovaries. After much testing, they discovered that the cells had actually originated in her fallopian tubes. They caught her ovarian cancer before it had actually gone to her ovaries!

Because of my mother's cancer history, I started getting yearly mammograms when I was thirty. Although I was being proactive, I wasn't ready to go the distance and take the BRCA gene test—a blood test that uses DNA analysis to identify harmful mutations in either one of the two breast cancer susceptibility genes—BRCA1 and BRCA2. That definitive test seemed way too scary, but, as it turned out, not as scary as being diagnosed with breast cancer in 2008, at age thirty-six.

Almost immediately afterwards, I had two lumpectomies and made plans to follow up with six weeks of radiation. It was between those two things that my doctor insisted I test for the BRCA gene. I relented and learned that I was BRCA-positive. Due to an eighty percent possibility of breast cancer recurrence in BRCA-positive women, my oncologist recommended a double mastectomy. Again, I relented. I was determined to get rid of any possible hiding place for those cancer cells.

Three years later, my daughter was born. Truly, if I thought my survival instincts were strong before she came into my life, they have been off the Richter scale since her arrival, which is why I now find myself contemplating removal of my tubes and ovaries. I've known for a while that having the BRCA gene (along with my mother's cancer history) puts me at a higher risk of contracting ovarian cancer at some point in my life, but I've been very resistant to an enforced menopause—partially due to the fact that my husband and I have yet to rule out having another child, and partially, well, because I don't want to deal with the symptoms of menopause. (Maybe it's time for me to read Dr. Sherry's Menopausal V chapter.) If I do decide to go the tube- and ovary-removal route, then I will definitely be looking to freeze some of my remaining eggs, if it's not too late.

If I've learned anything from my experience, it's that you can never ask too many questions. I went into research mode from the moment of my diagnosis and have remained there since. I ask questions and I maintain as healthy a lifestyle as possible—for me that means a vegetarian diet loaded with high alkaline foods and greens. It also means keeping stress to an absolute minimum; and did I mention asking tons of questions? Stay informed, stay healthy, and stay calm.

—Christina Applegate Actress

Given her mother's history of breast cancer, Christina knew she had a high risk for genetically linked breast cancer and made sure to have routine mammograms starting when she was thirty years old. Since she had extremely dense breasts her doctor decided to order a breast MRI, which is more sensitive in detecting breast cancer. At thirty-six years, her routine mammogram was negative but the follow up MRI done a few months later showed abnormal cancer cells, leading to an early diagnosis of breast cancer. Christina went on to test positive for the BRCA1 gene. Women like Christina have a sixty percent possibility of getting ovarian cancer given this genetic predisposition.

Christina has since founded Right Action for Women (www.rightactionforwomen.org) a non-profit foundation dedicated to educating women about what it means to be "high risk" for breast cancer and to supporting appropriate breast screening. The foundation also provides financial assistance to cover the costs of breast cancer screenings.

In sharing her own personal story, Christina hopes to empower women who are at a high risk for genetically linked breast cancer. Her call to fight is one she makes every day, through her foundation and through embracing loved ones and making each day count!

Preserving Fertility in Young Cancer Patients

In the U.S. alone, 1.7 million women cancer survivors were younger than forty at the age of diagnosis. At the time of their diagnoses, many of these young victims were not even thinking about family planning. Obviously, their first and foremost thoughts were of survival! But the truth is that many cancer treatments cause sterility—meaning that the ovaries cannot produce viable eggs—which puts an end to any chance of having a biological family. Enter: **Oocyte cryopreservation,** the process by which eggs are removed from the ovaries and frozen for future use.

For a young cancer patient, "there is a 40 to 50 percent chance of a live birth with either frozen eggs or frozen embryos," explains Dr. Nicole Noyes, MD, a professor and director of reproductive surgery at the New York University School of Medicine. In fact, many fertility experts think it is better to freeze *embryos*, which have a higher pregnancy rate than eggs. Of course, the big dilemma faced is that a young woman must use a known or unknown sperm donor—I mean, how many single women facing a cancer diagnosis at twenty-five can guess who their thirty-five or forty-year-old self may want to father their child? For that reason, counsel for young women in the area of fertility preservation is invaluable and essential during such a stressful time. Beating cancer and the prospect of having a future family need not be divergent goals!

Oncofertility is the newly created field of medicine that bridges oncology and reproductive research to explore and expand options for the reproductive future of cancer survivors. For the 140,000 women and men in their reproductive years who are diagnosed with cancer each year, oncofertility is a field providing revolutionary fertility hope. For women cancer survivors, another option, aside from using one's frozen eggs or embryos, is to use another women's eggs with their partner. If the plan includes carrying the baby herself, a cycle of IVF is called for. Alternately, many cancer survivors may use a surrogate to carry a pregnancy.

Unfortunately, the price of future family planning may seem out of reach to many. In order to proceed through just one cycle to harvest eggs and then put them on ice, the cost is around $10,000–$12,000. For this reason, there are a number of charity groups who will help young women with these seemingly insurmountable costs.

An Afterward…with Children

In my estimation, a happy-ever-after-early-cancer is a young woman who can, indeed, have the child she's always wanted. But there may be other issues, however non-life-threatening, that can present themselves after successful treatment for a cancer diagnosis.

Lani, a longtime friend and patient, was diagnosed with early breast cancer, DCIS—the most common type of non-invasive breast cancer—when she was thirty-nine. Her contagious joy and energy rarely waned, even after the diagnosis, because she knew that if one was to have breast cancer, DCIS was the most treatable, especially if caught early on. At the time, she was a single woman who knew she'd one day want a family. After her treatment, she went through intrauterine insemination using a donor sperm. Within two months she was pregnant, and after nine months of a thankfully uneventful pregnancy she delivered Charlie, a beautiful baby boy.

> "Having been diagnosed with DCIS and undergone a double mastectomy with full reconstruction in 2009, I am officially a breast cancer survivor. I consider myself more than a survivor though—I am a warrior. And now I am a mother. Not being able to breastfeed Charlie, I am eternally grateful to those moms who are donating milk to me to give Charlie the best start possible. I am related to one, dear friend's with another, and a stranger (though not anymore) to the third. There are more and more women like myself every day that are starting their families after having won some very hard battles. I figured it was time to stand proud and to share my gratitude. To give love and to receive... this is the greatest gift of life." —*Lani Shipman*

Unable to breast feed with her own breast milk, Lani instead used The Mother's Milk Bank, www.mothersmilk. com, to breastfeed Charlie for the first nine months of his life. Many breast cancer survivors, like Lani, who have had double mastectomies, experience the urgency to give their babies the breast milk they feel is necessary for sustenance in the first year of life. To that end, The Mother's Milk Bank is an amazing non-profit human milk bank dedicated to providing that sustenance and support.

Past Fifty and a Survivor

I hate to break the Pink V down into before and after fifty, as there is a great deal of overlap of emotional and physical issues regardless of age, but since fertility is obviously not an issue for the past fifty woman and her vagina, the biggest issues are emotional ones. After a cancer diagnosis (and treatment) this group of women tends to suffer from depression, anxiety, negative self-esteem, and sexual insecurities. The physical changes to sexual organs caused by chemotherapy, radiation, and the inability to be on estrogen therapy create the perfect trifecta of vaginal shut down. Since a whopping forty percent of women older than fifty do not have a sexual partner, the thought of getting out there in the dating world or on the newest dating app is daunting, at best.

Certain sexual difficulties and dysfunctions result from the physical and emotional issues caused by cancer. They include:

* Low sexual desire: disinterest in sex.
* Sexual aversion: an avoidance of any genital contact either by the survivor or her partner.
* Orgasmic dysfunction: absence or delay of orgasm.
* Vaginismus: spasm of the vaginal muscles, resulting in constriction of the vaginal opening and the prevention of vaginal penetration.
* Dyspareunia: painful intercourse.

The first step in seeking treatment for the not-so-pink V is to establish a trusted bond (and thereby an open communication) with your oncologist and gynecologist. Counseling with and without your partner is ideal as you navigate each hurdle in dealing with your cancer and the psychosexual issues that present themselves. Low sexual desire and sexual aversion can be addressed successfully through therapy and creative medical treatments, which may include antidepressants and anti-anxiety medication. Sometimes it's necessary for medication just to bring you back to an even keel and a sense of calm in order to address the physical issues.

Educate yourself on the effects of cancer along with asking your healthcare providers difficult question. This education will help you to embrace the treatment options for vaginal dysfunction. And there *are* treatment options: vaginal dilators, lubricants, topical lidocaine and estrogen therapy (if allowable), non-hormonal alternatives such as Osphena, the Mona Lisa Touch Laser, extra virgin coconut oil, and cannabis cream. The Mona Lisa is a game changer for many cancer survivors looking for a safe, effective and non-medicated treatment for vaginal dryness. **VVL**

Discuss these options with your oncologist to ensure the safety of your treatments. *Ask* whether estrogen-containing medications are okay. Remember that Osphena and herbal supplements often contain phytoestrogens, which are plant-derived compounds that are weaker than estrogen hormones, but nonetheless contain some estrogen.

Acceptance of your changing circumstances is crucial. Be honest about your fears and needs, and please communicate them with your doctor and partner. There is an appropriate treatment plan for you, one that will work best for you (and your partner).

Seek out support from groups with similar concerns to your own. The cancer support community is family unlike any you will ever experience. No matter where you are in the world, in your life, in your prognosis, there is a support group that can bring you energy and hope.

Cancer is not the end of your sexual health. It's a beginning of another chapter. You may have a healthy sexual life if you educate yourself on what to expect and if you fully explore your treatment options with your doctor and those you love. You deserve a healthy sex life, no matter the health hurdles, no matter the unforeseen circumstances that befall us in this wild, unwieldy, emotional journey we call life. The Pink V says FUCK CANCER!

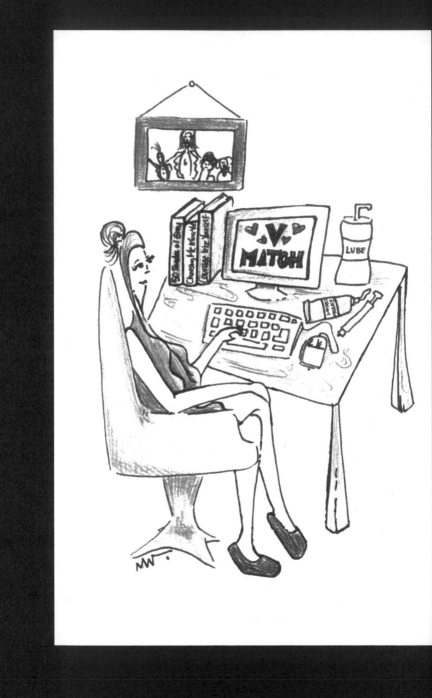

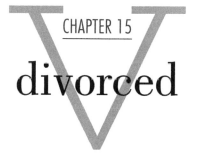

CHAPTER 15

divorced

“ New sex, new woman.
Nobody who is having great sex with her partner suddenly
divorces. In my case, my mate and I shared a bed for years after we
shared intimacies. When we divorced, I had been with only one man
for thirty years and the prospect of being with a new partner, let alone
finding one, was terrifying to me.

I was in my fifties, had birthed four kids, gone through menopause
and found my first gray pubic hair by the time we parted. Not only
that, but my self-confidence had been obliterated. Not his fault, really;
rather I'd long ago stopped thinking of myself as anyone other than
part of a duo. Who knew what *I* liked or wanted anymore? I hadn't
asked myself that question in a quarter of a century.

And what did *they*, the dateable men of the world, want and like?
Was anal now on the daily menu, as opposed to a Special? Oh God,
and blowjobs? Did I have to deal with that old dragon again? And

what about grooming down there? I'd kept tidy around my bikini lines, but I hadn't ever considered a "cut and color" to apply to my vagina as well as my head. When I asked around, I was introduced to a cottage industry of pubic hair coloring (hot pink!) and elimination as well as va-dazzling, where one artfully applies crystals and beads with Crazy Glue to their bush-business.

It made my neck ache just looking down there long enough to take stock of it all. Still, I suspected that vaginal grooming, to quote a great Alaskan, would be "like putting lipstick on a pig" if my vagina was too tired to satisfy a man. After having my babies, I'd always asked my O.B. to stitch things back up snugly, but I wondered if that just meant that the "barn door" was small, while the barn, itself, was cavernous and full of spider webs and dust. When I asked him for an honest appraisal he sanely replied, "Don't do anything because you don't even know the size of the new penises you might meet." Funny how I'd completely forgotten that it could be "the meat" as well as "the motion."

I had no idea that the prize for surviving divorce and finding the right new partner was the delirious, mind-bending and unexpected joy of New Sex! The kind of sex where kissing is sustained and urgent. Where feeling a hand move up my back to release my bra is unbearably erotic and the feeling of new hands touching me fills me with anticipation and wonder. This just isn't talked about enough in divorce conversations.

Well, at least until Dr. Sherry wrote this book. We've been friends for almost twenty years and yet I felt slightly perverse discussing how obsessed I was by sex at this time in my life. *She-ology* reminded me that my V is as much a part of me as my heart and my brain and that it will stay a vibrant organ as long as the other two. And if it's the last one to go, lucky me!

The chance to be discovered all over again as I am now and yet to feel like I did when I was twenty transformed me. Divorce wasn't the end of me, but rather the beginning of my next journey. I almost hate to talk about it to still-married friends because it's like describing a meal at the French Laundry to people on a gluten-free diet, but it's spectacular. I reclaimed a huge part of me that I'd forgotten existed when I became this new sexual being and I'm still cherishing it every day.

—Vicki Iovine Author, Attorney

Carol, a 52-year-old patient, recently divorced her husband of twenty-five years. They'd both known for a while that that it was coming, but they waited until the kids were in college and out of the house. Carol went on Match.com and relished all "winks" she got from prospective beaus. It was no wonder she received so much attention; a perfect size eight in tight jeans and low cut blouses revealing brand new cleavage, she'd also recently had her eyes "done" by a Hollywood plastic surgeon to the stars. Sexy and effusive, she seemed the perfect catch for that age-appropriate guy. But, as she confessed during our appointment, she was worried about life after divorce. She hadn't had sex with anyone (but herself) for ten years. She was terrified to go on a date or even think about having sex again, and so she asked me what she needed to know in order to navigate the dating world at her age—and in 2017—because she was ready, and willing, to get it right the second time around.

You and your more-than-likely-neglected vagina are about to go out and meet the world for the first time in years. Whether you're reeling from your divorce or doing cartwheels out of your lawyer's office, it's a major transition time on many fronts: emotional, psychological, financial. But nothing causes more anxiety (or anticipation) than the prospect of taking your vagina out for a spin after the abandonment that often accompanies the final years of an unraveling marriage.

You're way beyond the blushing teenager you may have been in your high school Sex Ed class. You've had a family, a career, years of hard-won experience and wisdom, and yet, here you are, hoping to find the pleasure and satisfaction you've been without for too long. According to recent studies the divorce rate for first marriages is fifty percent; for second marriages it's sixty percent; and for third marriages it's seventy-three percent. And so, this large pool of newly single, middle-aged women (and men) may be more in need of a good Sex Ed talk than any other population in our culture. Teenagers certainly know where to look online for info about and exposure to sex (another conversation entirely, addressed fully in the Tween V, Chapter 2).

The realities of being a single, sexually active adult are very different than they were in past decades. There's a lot to learn and, when the time is right, *discuss* with a new partner. The rules have changed in 2017, as have the necessary conversations that accompany the start of any kind of relationship. Sexual activity can mean health risks, and so dating etiquette is not just about who pays for dinner or how many dates it's proper to have before going to bed with your new friend. It's more about when to have that uncomfortable conversation about sexual history and whether your partner has any sexually transmitted diseases. While the good news may be that you don't have to worry about getting pregnant, you can still be on the receiving end of a number of STDs. And because, YES, you do have to use a condom every time, that's a part of the new dialogue about sex as well.

Communication is Key

Dee, a vibrant, gorgeous, and hilarious 73-year-old patient of mine recently started dating again after her husband of thirty-five years passed away. She was so excited to share how she'd met "an amazing, magical man" through the Santa Monica Hiking Club. She saw great humor in her official role as "cougar," since her new boyfriend was fifteen years her junior, and she couldn't help but regale me with tales of her newfound sexual passion. She was having sex at least twice a day, and her orgasms had never been better. She and her young stud of a boyfriend had even started working their way through the book 365 Sex Positions, and she told me about sexual positions I hadn't even heard of. It was wonderful to see Dee's enjoyment in life and love at the age of seventy-three.

Sounds great, right? So why was she paying a visit to my office? Dee and her boyfriend had been dating for nine months, and she'd just noticed something on her vagina that she'd never seen before. By the time I saw her she'd had pain and itching for four days. I already suspected the cause from her vivid description, but of course I proceeded with an exam, just to be certain.

I found a group of ulcerative lesions (sores) that I eventually diagnosed as Herpes Simplex virus type 2. When I told Dee, she was shocked and mortified. Her new beau had never disclosed any sexually transmitted diseases. When she told him about her diagnosis, he did *then* mention that he'd had herpes on his penis in the past, but it had been a very long time since his last outbreak. Obviously this was information that would have served her much better *before* they'd had sexual contact. **VVL**

Fortunately, Dee and her "magical man" were able to overcome this uncomfortable surprise revelation. They're still together today and maintain a much more open discussion of their sex lives and relationship than ever before. Dee definitely didn't take the easy route to get to this deeper connection, as she'll now carry the herpes virus with her for the rest of her life. If her partner had told her he had HSV from the outset, he could have been put on a medication, prophylactically, to prevent him from having a herpes outbreak. Safe for him. Safe for her.

Now I know it's easy to wag your fingers and imagine doing it differently, but this patient is actually quite typical of people who are entering the dating world and becoming sexually active for the first time in decades. Many are naïve about the realities. Some want to have a frank discussion with new partners but chicken out at the last minute. So here's some tough love. Recent studies prove what I frequently see in my office, which might shock you:

* The rate of STIs in those over the age of forty-five has doubled.
* One in five sexually active singles reported using condoms regularly. Only twelve percent of men and thirty-two percent of women said they used one every time.
* Those over the age of forty-five had the lowest rate of condom use.
* Older immune systems are less effective at fighting infections, which can increase the risk of STIs.
* Older women have less natural lubrication and thinning vaginal tissue, leading to tears, which then create a higher risk of transmitting STIs.

* The number of older people diagnosed with HIV has nearly doubled. Fifteen percent of new diagnoses of HIV were in people past the age of fifty.
* Delays in diagnosis and treatment are more common in the older population, allowing infections to become more advanced and harder to treat.

Intimidated? Don't be. For starters, you're not alone. As mentioned already, this population is fast growing, and everyone's feeling pretty much the same way. Recent studies also show that sex is not an easy topic for ANYONE to discuss with their healthcare providers, and so there are lots of other women (and men) out there who are nervously facing the facts. Talking to your doctor is a great way to ease into the conversation and gain valuable knowledge. Hey, if you've got to practice saying the words VAGINA and STI out loud a few times before saying it to your date, who's a better guinea pig then your gynecologist, right?

During your routine gynecologic exam—which you should definitely undergo before you become sexually active, and have regularly once you are sexually active—your healthcare provider should get a complete sexual history from you, along with routine STI cultures. This conversation should include a refresher on the true definition of safe sex.

It's sometimes a good idea for new partners to be tested together, so they receive their results at the same time as a part of becoming closer. This approach might be another way for you to handle the STI situation. *Hey, why don't we get a drink...and a test?* Just a thought.

How DO You Practice Safe Sex?

Melissa, a newly divorced patient with a stunning Saks Fifth Avenue wardrobe and exhaustive knowledge of the best New Zealand Sauvignon Blancs, recently asked, "Do I need to have my new boyfriend wear a condom when I give him a blow job?" Melissa went on to say that she'd never liked giving blow jobs to her ex-husband because he had a crooked tip. But, excluding her ex, she loved giving head and even liked to swallow. She just had concerns about her "future on the job," she joked. Because most women can barely bring themselves to talk about blowjobs, let alone admit that it's their favorite thing about sex, I so appreciated Melissa's candor. It was just a matter of keeping her safe.

I know it's not sexy. And this information may be hard to swallow. (Ba-dum-bum). But the correct answer is, "Yes, you do need to use a condom during blow jobs!" This is the only way to know you're less likely to get HPV in the back of your throat. Also, remember this: having sores in your mouth or open sours on your genitals when you are exposed to a man's ejaculate, or a woman's vaginal fluid, can increase your risk of getting HIV if your new partner has this virus. Just because HIV is not grabbing headlines the way it did a decade ago does not mean this terrifying virus has gone away. Protect and educate yourself and your partners.

It can be hard to know how to even begin a conversation about sex, especially if you're coming out of a long-term relationship that didn't include any, and you've got a new partner in your life for the first time in years—or decades. So here's what I've gleaned from my time in the trenches with my patients: First of all, I do not think this topic is good pillow talk. The words don't always come out right to begin with, and, on top of that, passion can interfere with your ability to speak or think clearly.

Because this is a serious topic, it should be addressed before you even get into the bedroom. This is not the same conversation as, "This is what I really like... touch me here." But, hopefully, if this conversation goes well, the conversation about what turns you on won't be far behind. On the other hand, this might not be something you want to bring up on the first date. Although, realistically, that's better than what often happens, which is to have a few cocktails on the first or second night out and then away you go, jumping right into bed before you've had time to get comfortable about anything, let alone the discussion of *prophylactics*. So I think the whole point is to slow it down and let everything unfold in a timely manner, with a sex talk at just the right time: BEFORE the sex happens.

It doesn't have to be all doom and gloom, though. This is an exciting moment for you—a transition time full of new experiences and pleasures. And taking an enlightened, empowered approach to your newly divorced vagina and your (safe) sex life can be a major component of taking a more active, confident role in getting and giving exactly what you want in the bedroom, which, let's be honest, will probably be a remarkable new turn of events coming at the end of an unhappy marriage or union.

Okay, so you're empowered. You're ready. Now, what do you actually say? Well, that depends completely on your personality. Some women are just out there. It could be as direct as: "What STIs have you had? And do you have multiple sexual partners?"

Or it could be something a lot subtler than that. I think the important thing is that no one wants to feel judged. And the more open and honest you can be, the more open and honest your date is likely to be in return. So you might want to skip something like, "Do you have the warts?" But that's *just* my professional opinion.

Okay, so what are we really dealing with here anyhow? It is crucial to talk about your previous sexual experiences and if there is a history of any sexually transmitted diseases on both sides. You should know the list and go over each of them: Human Papilloma Virus (HPV), Chlamydia, Gonorrhea, Herpes Simplex virus on the genitals and the mouth, Tricho-moniasis, Hepatitis B and C, and Human Immunodeficiency virus (HIV).

The human papilloma virus (HPV) is the most commonly passed STI. Condoms do not provide complete protection against HPV transmission. So that's the one that's got me most concerned these days. Not to mention that HPV is the most common sexually transmitted infection, affecting eighty to ninety percent of men and women, and causing genital warts, cervical and oral cancers. Your risk of exposure is directly related to the number of sexual partners you've had. The more partners you and your sexual partner have had, the higher your risk of being exposed to HPV. The good news: there's a vaccine. The bad news: it's only recommended for those between the ages of eleven and twenty-six who are at the beginning of their sexual lives (which is why we address HPV with greater nuance in **Benched V,** Chapter 12). The vaccine is ideal for those who haven't been exposed to any of the big 9 high-risk types of HPV, which translates to those women who have never had *any* sexual contact.

But what about a *renewed* sexual life? Shouldn't a divorced woman get the HPV vaccine? It's clear more studies are needed in the older age groups, but I definitely think it's worth having a conversation with your healthcare provider to consider the vaccination. Many of my patients opt to get the vaccine just in case there is some protection from this epidemic and contagious virus. Being pro-active and asking these tough questions are part of empowering you and your V in this next chapter in life.

Getting Your Divorced V Ready for Its Close Up

So, you found a partner, you were courageous enough to have "the talk," and now it's time. What should you expect? Well, for starters, things have changed since you first had sex with your ex, and not only in terms of the realities of being sexually active today, which we've already discussed. Your body is different, and so is that of your new partner.

The aging process affects men and women differently (and we fully address the specific issues faced by women in the Mature V, Chapter 6). Women tend to have less lubrication as they age, combined with obstacles associated with menopause and the loss of estrogen. Vaginal dryness is more the norm than not after age fifty. Women should never be afraid to use a lubricant or even a sex toy, such as a vibrator, to help make your sexual experience pleasurable. The mature vagina might also need some additional estrogen to avoid the changes associated with low estrogen, including delicate, dry and fragile vaginal tissue, which can result in tearing, burning, and pain during sex, and allow easy access for STIs. Taking time to educate yourself and care for your vagina properly before you start dating again can go far toward enhancing your enjoyment, which hopefully will be a part of enhancing your partner's pleasure, too. **VVL**

You're not alone, and it's not only your fellow ladies who are facing the realities of getting older. Men are also dealing with their own sexual issues related to aging. Life stressors can play a role in the bedroom for both genders. There are overlapping topics that need to be discussed in a supportive and honest way. Again, being comfortable with your partner starts with an open and transparent conversation, with your clothes on. The bedroom just isn't the ideal place to have these sensitive discussions. Have the talk early, so you can enjoy yourselves later.

What's Up with the Treatment for Male Erectile Dysfunction?

For most men, the plumbing does not work as well, or as quickly, over time. Medical problems and medication side effects can also contribute to sexual difficulties. Whatever the cause, the inability to maintain an erect penis for sex and intimacy is called erectile dysfunction (ED) and happens to men typically after the age of fifty, especially those who have prostate cancer, diabetes, high blood pressure, and heart disease. Certain medications used for depression, anxiety and other medical conditions can create or worsen ED.

Culturally, we tend to think of ED as a problem because it can lead to an inability to have intercourse. However, there's another whole factor you should be aware of before you go to bed with a man with ED, which can lead to the painful circumstances my patient faced. The most common treatment for ED is what we commonly refer to as "the little blue pill," or Viagra, which creates a hard, long lasting erection. Just what the man wants. And exactly what the woman with an extra-sensitive, post-menopausal vagina does *not* want slamming into her dehydrated and delicate vagina.

So, if you're dating a new man, it's not just a good idea to have a frank conversation about STDs, it can also be helpful to find out if he has ED, so you'll know what kind of intercourse to expect. In addition to oral medications, such as Viagra, some men treat their ED with other methods such as a penile suppository inserted into the penis before sex, an injection at the base of the penis, a vacuum that helps maintain a penile erection, or a penile implant that can be inflated during sex. Eastern options include herbs and supplements.

As any ED treatment could soon be a part of your sex life, having an open, supportive conversation can help to make the experience more pleasurable for both partners. And always remember this: ED can create a lot of anxiety, frustration and stress, not only for the man but also for his partner. For optimal success, the decision on what treatment option to use for ED should be a conversation involving both partners. I also suggest involving a therapist so you and your partner both feel supported during this challenging time.

Divorced, Not Done

Let's be real: being single over the age of forty is difficult. In general, women beyond forty years are most unhappy when it comes to dating. They often feel helpless, and this can be accompanied by some depression and frustration at finding themselves without a really good pool of eligible men (or women) to date. Plus, dating just gets more challenging as you get older. Not to mention that divorced women have often gained weight during their marriages or following the birth of their children, so they don't always feel very confident or sexy.

My most heartfelt and challenging conversations occur during an examination of a Divorced V. Women entering the difficult post-divorce chapters are usually focused on everything except themselves. If they were protective of their kids before, they may become wolf-like in their focus and protection after the divorce, with the thought of dating seeming like a faraway fantasy. My best friend who divorced spent the first year crying nightly and sharing horror stories of her failed marriage egged on by her favorite Two-Buck-Chuck cabernet. When the New Year rolled around I bought her a membership to a cycling gym. At first she said there was no way she could make that kind of commitment to a bicycle seat, but when I told her she could burn up to 700 calories in a 45-minute workout she said, "Hmmm, let me re-think how efficient forty-five minutes of a workout could be at burning three glasses of wine," and she accepted my gift. Weekly cycle workouts turned into a 15-pound weight loss, a healthier diet, restriction of her wine intake to Fridays and Saturdays (and a two drink maximum) and membership on the dating website Zoosk. com. My best friend is currently dating an age-appropriate guy, and she thanks me every day for taking the time to "kick [her] ass back into reality." New beginnings are created when *you* are at the helm.

Those of us who have been through the roller coaster ride of divorce know that reflection and introspection happen once the clouds have lifted. With time and patience, you will find strength, resilience, and new beginnings. What most divorced women ultimately realize is that happiness is essential to healing. Try not to be too hard on yourself. Take care of your-self. Enjoy pleasures where they come. Ultimately you are the only person that can make it happen.

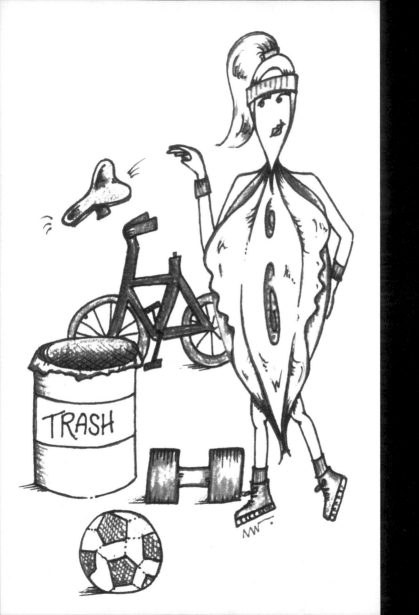

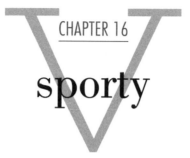

CHAPTER 16

sporty

"My bike is my best friend, but my bike seat can be a thorn in my side, specifically, a pain in my Sporty V.

I ride road bikes for fun now, after years of competitive racing. When I first started racing I was warned: It's a dangerous sport. It's not a matter of *if* you crash; it's a matter of *when*.

But no one prepared me for the other, *hidden* dangers of cycling. [Cue ominous music.] The dreaded painful V. Seriously, there's nothing worse.

Most weekends you would find me racing, which meant 15–20 hours of weekly training, with an average ride of 2.5 hours—some weekend rides went 4 or 5 hours. That's a lot of time perched on a hard carbon-fiber saddle the width of a small postcard.

The last half hour of a long ride was mostly spent wriggling around from side to side, sliding from front to back and lifting up and down in an attempt to find a comfortable position—anything to relieve the pressure on Sporty V. Even a specially designed cutout seat—one favored by most male and female riders—didn't always help me with the V blues.

Showering after a training ride was agony. The hit of hot water on an area that had taken a marathon beating was akin to putting lemon juice on a cut. I'll admit most of my suffering was due to my lack of preparation before a ride. I was always in too much of a hurry to take the simplest precautions.

In short order, here are steps you can take to alleviate the pressure on your delicate V and minimize damage.

- Find a good Chamois cream, like "Beljum Budder," which you'll slather inside your padded shorts before your ride. This is one time you won't want to go *light on the budder*!
- Maintain a bikini wax—smooth as a baby, no hair no tear.
- When you are done with your ride, don't sit around in your cycling shorts. Shower and then let your pummeled parts air-dry. Walk around naked as long as you can to give your poor Sporty V the freedom it deserves.
- Finally, take heed of Dr. Sherry's tips on the Sporty V! She's on spot in providing pertinent information for women who spin, bike, and horseback ride. You might even feel encouraged to take that first ride, whatever it's on.

Remember, V also stands for Victory.

—Louise Keoghan TV Producer & Director

Sporty V

Twenty-eight-year-old Bren, a triathlete, could be the poster girl for health and wellness. She even dresses the part, looking like she's just stepped out of a photo shoot for Fabletics workout clothes. As exhausted as I was just hearing about the rigorous training schedule for her latest competition, she was excited and confident, except for one small detail. "You know, Dr. Sherry, I love training, I love it all," she said, "and I have no problems with the running and swimming, but the biking has been really, really hard on my lady parts... I can't even feel them, I'm so numb down there after biking. Seriously, what can I do? I mean my clit gets so sore that I can't even have sex. What do I do?!"

It's a subject that gets little attention, but affects countless women: Many women face problems related to cycling, spinning, and horseback riding that can be traumatizing to the vagina. Up until recent times women were often discouraged from participating in these particular activities because of vaginal maladies that seemed unavoidable. Of course we know now that there are ways to avoid trauma to the vagina, but some women, unlike Bren, are either too embarrassed to ask the right questions or they imagine that they must simply grin and bear the pain.

It's estimated that nineteen million women regularly participate in cycling or spinning as their primary source of physical exercise. That's a whole lot of potential vaginal trauma. For triathlon competitors, the longest distance is also covered by bicycle. There's V-trauma on top of the potential muscle pain and cramps of the swimming and running segments. Many of my patients participate in the AIDS ride each year, a week long, 550-mile bike ride from San Francisco to Los Angeles to raise money and awareness for HIV/AIDS.

Averaging eighty miles a day, these peerless women riders take a beating not only in the usual places that the men do (calves, thighs, arms, etc.), they have the added injustice of chafing, numbness, pain, swelling and, often, abscesses in the area of their vaginas. The more experienced women riders in the group not only understand "pacing," they know that there are ways to protect their vaginas. Less common are the complaints that women have due to injuries suffered in horseback riding—those complaints being less common only because cyclists far outnumber riders, especially in my practice—but the problems and injuries are similar.

Professor Luc Baeyons, a gynecologist who specializes in sports medicine, found that numbness, skin infections, chronic swelling, and lymphatic damage are the most common complaints amongst female cyclists. Sixty percent of Dr. Baeyons study group reported *some* degree of genital discomfort. Because of the way the vagina is positioned on a bicycle seat there is an unfamiliar pressure on the delicate soft tissue of the labia majora and minora, better known as the lips of the vagina. On a prolonged bicycle ride, pressure on the tailbone, lower back and groin restricts blood flow and increases skin irritation, resulting in vaginal numbness—especially in the area of the clitoris—genital pain and/or reduced genital sensation. These problems may also result from spinning and horseback riding.

Other problems associated with cycling, spinning, and riding include vaginal infections such as yeast and bacterial due to the moisture buildup from poor vaginal ventilation that occurs with these sports. Constant pressure can also bring about cysts, although **recumbent cycling** tends not to create the same problems with the vagina that upright cycling causes, since pressure is transferred to the buttocks instead of the vagina. **VVL**

You might be thinking by now that it's a wonder any of us dare to incorporate these sports into our daily activities, but there are, of course, things you can do to minimize injury (and insult) to your vagina if your passion is, indeed, cycling, spinning or horseback riding. Which brings us to:

Safe Riding Tips for Your Riding V

* **Appropriate Saddle Selection:** If you're participating in prolonged periods of cycling/spinning—meaning thirty or more minutes a pop—it is of utmost importance to invest in a comfortable bicycle seat. One of the best is made by Selle Italia SMP, but shop around and ask your other cycling enthusiast friends what they're sitting on. There are also gel seat covers especially made for spin bikes, which can help in your more stationary exercises, since typical bike seats at the local gym are not really vagina-friendly. Be proactive and bring your own seat cover when you spin at the gym!

* **Cycling Shorts:** These are not just for fashion, although you might not know it from all the hipster cycling enthusiasts stopping by Starbucks on a Sunday afternoon. Padded cycling shorts are a must since they truly do provide protection to your most sensitive areas. Cycling shorts are actually meant to be worn without underwear, providing a snug fit to avoid the friction brought on by loose-fitting shorts. Avoid shorts with a weave, woven texture, or synthetic

and raised threading as those things promote tears, friction and seam burns in all the wrong female places. Always wash your cycling shorts after each ride. Some fabulous brands of padded cycling shorts include: Assos F1 Mile, SheBeest, and OEM. Serious riders spend nearly as much money on these Maseratis of padded shorts as they do on their bicycles, believing that it is worth every penny, especially on rides longer than a couple hours.

* **Topical Creams:** Certain emollient creams can be applied to the vaginal area and upper thighs to help prevent chronic skin irritations such as chafing, rashes and itching. A few brands I'd recommend are Assos Chamois Cream, Udderly Smooth, Hoo-Haa Cream, and Rapha's chamois cream. To bring relief from yeast infections, the anti-fungal over-the-counter cream clotrimizole 1% combined with corn starch (in place of talcum powder) is a good bet. And Vaseline is a great, inexpensive go-to protectant from friction and chafing.

* **Professional Bike Fit:** Find a bike professional to fit your bike in proportion to your height. Believe me, proper bicycle height in relation to your body will help prevent injury. A professional can help you adjust your bike stem and handles to your cycling style as well. It's recommended that your bike stem and handles be fixed in a way that sets your posture at a sixty-degree angle to horizontal position, which brings us to...

* **Proper Cycling Posture:** Dr. Frank Sommer, a German urologist and sports medicine specialist,

found that posture greatly affects the pressure on your genitals, which, in turn, affects the genital blood supply. The more stretched out you are on your bike, the less pressure is put on the soft tissue and the less chance of sexual health problems. As per Dr. Sommer's findings, a cyclist riding a bike with her body at thirty degrees to horizontal may experience up to a seventy percent reduction in blood supply to the genitals. So keep that posture at the sixty degree angle.

* **Post Ride Activity:** Following that long ride, a warm bath with Aveeno bath powder is not only the most relaxing reward you can give yourself, this little luxury increases blood flow to the vagina and moisturizes the skin. Never drive home in your sweaty shorts after a long bike ride; change into a clean, dry pair until you can jump in the shower. I always have antiseptic feminine wet wipes along for a ride. They're a great way to clean and soothe your vagina after a long ride in those fitted shorts.

* **Vaginal Hygiene:** During an extended bicycle ride moisture builds up in the vaginal area preventing proper ventilation and allowing an increased risk for yeast and bacterial infections and other skin ailments. When you have a chance it's important to shower, or, at least, to clean the vagina. It's preferable that you change into looser, less restrictive clothing as well. This will allow for increased blood flow to the vagina and for decompression in the area. And while we're addressing the V, the question is: To shave or not to shave? The consensus seems to be not to shave the pubic hairs but to trim the area so that the hair serves

as a cushion. Avoid long cycling rides during your menstrual period, but if you *are* riding, be aware that the string of a tampon can also cause irritation to the vaginal tissue. Cleaning the vagina with non-fragrant soap can help prevent cysts, acne, and other skin-related infections.

Although the sports of cycling and horseback riding seem to present the greatest potential for V injury, there are a couple other activities that can also cause distress.

Waterskiing V

Ever been waterskiing? Then you probably know what a water enema feels like! On the other side of things (literally) water spraying into the vagina, better known as a waterskiing douche, can be equally painful and uncomfortable. Since waterskiing usually involves speeds of about thirty miles per hour, a fall may not only be terrifying, it can be quite dangerous. The force of such a fall can lead to lacerations to the vagina, perineum, and rectum either from hitting the water's surface, or worse, from hitting a waterski or wakeboard. Severe bleeding, pain, and infections can develop if vaginal lacerations go untreated. If you waterski, especially if you're a novice, it's important to not only be aware of your form, but to know *how to fall*. Like any other sport that takes skill and practice, work with someone who knows what they're doing. Other water activities involving high speeds include wake boarding, jet skiing and the simple (but fun) ride of being pulled behind a boat on an inner tube, all of which can all cause vaginal injuries. Wear protective swim pants, and boat with experienced friends to help avoid injury to your Water Sporty V.

Swimming V

First off, according to statistics, we love to swim. Swimming ranks number three in popularity of sports activities, and, according to PHIT America, number two in the growth of top activities, with 3.1 million new participants in 2013. You can do it at three or ninety-three. It's the total body workout, no tools or toys or special equipment (aside from a pool) necessary. For inspiration, one needs to look no further than long-distance swimmer and sports journalist Diana Nyad, who, in 2013, at age sixty-four, became the first person to swim 110 miles from Havana, Cuba, to Key West, Florida without the aid of a shark cage.

You may have already surmised that a lot of my patients swim. Some *love* to swim, and some do it dutifully, but they do it with purpose and conviction. Whether they're doing it as play or sport, I'm frequently asked about whether or not chlorine affects the vagina, and although chlorine does act to clean out bacteria and other nasty germs found in a swimming pool, it generally shouldn't be a problem for the vagina. The real problem usually caused by chlorine is skin dryness. Anyone who has spent a few hours in a swimming pool can tell you this. But as far as the water itself from an ocean or pool affecting your vagina, any problems usually stem from infections caused by wearing a wet bathing suit for a long period of time once you are *out* of the water. Think of it (for a second) in terms of marinating in a chlorine or saltwater wash. See what I mean?

Best way to avoid any problems from swimming or water play is to take off your bathing suit and jump into some dry clothing.

Sex on the Beach
(and I Don't Mean the Cocktail)

Nineteen-year-old Allie is the quintessential Southern California gal. She bikes, she swims, she surfs, she has fun no matter where she is or what she's doing, which includes sex—lots of it apparently. Even after all the wild stories I hear from my patients, sometimes Allie can actually make me blush when she talks about some of the crazy places she "hooks up" with her boyfriend. On this particular visit, she told me that they were planning a trip to Cancun, Mexico and they'd fantasized about having sex in the ocean. "Would it be safe?" She asked.

Well, sex in the ocean certainly might seem like a perfect fantasy to some, especially if Bora Bora is your backdrop, but the truth is that ocean sex would not necessarily be more ideal than a tumble in a dirt bath. Between the sand, floating trash, oil spills, toxic chemicals, sewage runoff, and other unwanted bacteria, ocean water is a cornucopia of potential vaginal infection and irritation. Saltwater pools may seem a safer bet for some water-world sexual play, but you still risk exposure to harmful chemicals and unwelcome bacteria. If you envision sex in the water, best to invite a friend into a nice, clean shower.

I encourage you: swim, bike, cycle, ride. Be active and find joy in your activities and sports. But just as your head needs a helmet for protection when you ride, your vagina needs protecting, too. Sporty V knows that the best offense is a good defense!

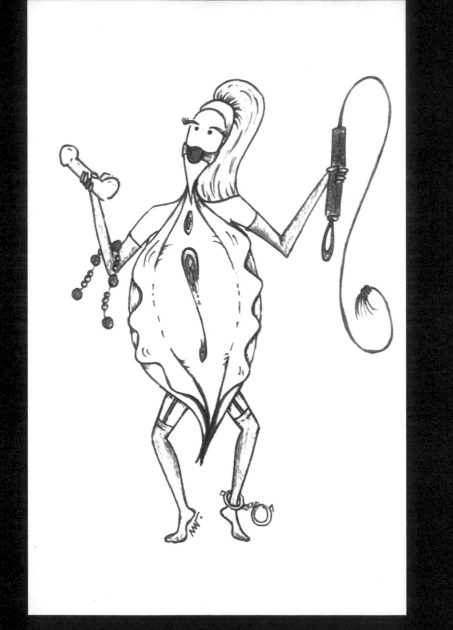

CHAPTER 17

adventurous

"Ohhhh...whooooaaaa...it's like a dark tunnel. There's this little opening, but then it has these walls and layers, and it's all pink and shiny. It's like a weird cave.

I didn't realize it at the time, but I was having my first gynecological exam by my best friend, Debbie Gerber. We were seven.

She was sleeping over, and after a night of "sneaking food"—which was basically raiding the refrigerator and cupboards for crap food and chocolate—we had settled into my canopy bed (with the pull out trundle) and were ready to *explore*. That's what we called it, exploring. Like Lewis and Clark on a great, unknown expedition, we were discovering and exploring our vaginas. That was my first adventure with my V. We really knew how to party then.

We were so innocent, curious and we were trying to figure out the vast mysteries and the meaning of this secret passageway within our little bodies. There was no shame, only questions and wonder.

She-ology

Many years later this would be known as "going to the gyno." There wasn't any chocolate, you had to pay, and it could be awkward and scary depending upon the "explorer." I remember my first; he was a kindly old doctor who would place his hands on my freshly grown breasts in examination and ask, "How're my boys?" To this day I can't decide if he was a bit pervy or slightly senile.

Fortunately for me, after a lot of searching, I discovered Dr. Sherry Ross, a gyno I could feel comfortable with. She's the kind of doctor who not only provides thoughtful answers to my questions, but she also creates an atmosphere where I feel comfortable in asking those questions—though, I'd like to suggest maybe hiding some "healthy" candy around the office so I might sneak some before the exam, in deference to the good old days in my canopy bed with Debbie Gerber.

My point is: Feeling comfortable in addressing your concerns and feeling free to ask questions is exactly how you ought to feel in any relationship. Whether your partner is a man or woman, robot or plant, you've got to feel comfortable. It helps to be secure in who you are. It's only when you are secure in your own sexuality, whatever that might be, and when you feel safe in your relationships that you can experiment, go out on a limb, and experience the fun, intimacy and excitement that you—all of us—deserve.

Happy exploring!

—Gina Gershon Actress

Adventurous V

Tiffany's been my "wild child" patient since I became her gynecologist seventeen years ago. Now forty-six, and a real estate agent in Malibu, she's as effervescent and entertaining as she is successful. A tall striking blond, with designer nails and a penchant towards the latest health trends, Tiffany always manages a two-hour, toxin-cleansing Bikram Yoga session and The Manhattan blow-out at Dry Bar, before her yearly Pap smear. She and her husband Tommy have been happily married for fourteen years—since meeting on a "singles only" vacation in Puerto Vallarta. As I've come to know Tiffany, and she's regaled me with stories of her and Tommy's rather voracious sexual appetites, she's come to know my mantra as "to each his own," so on her past visit, when she asked my opinion of "Swinging," I didn't bat an eye. Tommy had asked her if she would be interested in attending the Malibu Swingers Club cocktail party for new members. (Frankly, I felt glaringly unhip to be so late to the table in learning that swinging was, pardon the pun, on an upswing!) Tiffany had far more concerns about STIs (sexually transmitted infections) than she did about an open sexual lifestyle, so it seemed a good time for a crash refresher course about hygiene, condoms, and sexually transmitted diseases, including HPV.

Open-minded, uninhibited, *adventurous*. Does that describe you and your V? Or maybe it reminds you of someone you know. Either way, it's important to know the advantages along with the disadvantages (and, sometimes, the risks) of sexual creativity, especially in the *extreme*. Then again, take away the judgment completely and the fact remains that what's extreme for one woman may be normal for another! I mean, some of us like to bike rustic shady roads, and some of us prefer extreme motocross. Know what I mean? Your V knows...

Swinging (or "What exactly does Swinging mean, and am I crazy for even considering it?")

Swinging in America (Now why hasn't anyone used that for a movie title yet?) has its roots in early 1950s upscale sub-urban communities. It was, and remains, a way for married couples to engage in recreational, non-monogamous relation-ships, ostensibly without cheating on each other. One married couple may look to the lifestyle as a chance to spice up their own sex life; another may be looking for the opportunity to explore bisexuality without being labeled as gay. A couple may be drawn to Swinging as a chance to act at voyeur, without the risk of being judged, and yet another may view Swinging as an antidote to divorce! Partners who might otherwise run the risk of sneaky (and, ultimately, hurtful or destructive) extramarital affairs may consider Swinging as an acceptable alternative. Whatever the reason, participants in this unique lifestyle are free to experience their sexuality outside of the fear or shame of what others may think, as, aside from acceptance, there are certain unwritten rules of privacy within the Swinging com-munity. And, no, you're not crazy for considering it.

Our sexuality is a natural and important part of our iden-tity, and it can be driven by a number of things, including our upbringing, religious convictions, friendships, past sexual experiences and self-confidence. If you and your partner are interested in exploring your sexuality through Swinging, you need to discuss the implications of such an endeavor before you embark on it.

Voice your concerns, fears or insecurities to each other, and, certainly, know that the use of condoms is standard operating procedure as the risk for STIs potentially increases with additional sexual partners, no matter your erotic preference.

When Three's Company

I can always count on Cassandra to arrive make-up perfect and dressed to the nines in one of her Plus Size designer outfits. A successful, charismatic 49-year-old, Cassandra is the type of woman anyone would want to befriend, so it wasn't surprising that Shannon, thirty-five and a newly transplanted Angeleno, had made overtures to Cassandra at their weekly Pilates class in Studio City. Over a three-hour coffee date, Cassandra bonded quickly with Shannon and her husband, Taylor. Over the course of six months, coffee dates turned into weekly dinners, which turned into Friday movie nights, and then regular sleepovers. At her check-up, Cassandra calmly and quite happily told me that she was in a wonderful and loving polyamorous relationship with the couple. She was an open part of their entire family. As I listened to Cassandra gush about her new family, I found I was having an internal conversation with myself: It's consensual, transparent and loving... I mean, what could possibly be wrong with that? She must have heard me thinking because she answered, "You know, Doctor Ross, I finally feel as though I am in an honest, completely transparent, and loving relationship." I think I did say, "Who can argue that logic?" At least I hope I said that out loud.

Polyamory

An adventurous, open love between committed partners, *polyamory* is a type of lifestyle that provides freedom in bringing another partner (or two...or five) to a relationship without boundaries or judgment. There are many happily committed couples that believe it's possible to love more than one person at a time, not just in the bedroom, but also in day-to-day life. Although I deem it adventurous, it's not as uncommon as you may think. In fact, as many as five percent of Americans are currently in a consensual, non-monogamous relationship, which means that the committed couple are allowed to look outside the relationship for love or sex or both. Traditional boundaries don't apply, and the rules are by mutual agreement. Obviously, this form of love sharing is for those of a similar mindset, those who are open to welcoming new partners to an existing relationship. Those involved in polyamory contend that this particular type of love is based on honesty, respect, and romantic commitment—of course, the basis for any good and satisfying relationship—but polys (as they're referred to) design their own rules as to what *their* poly family ought to look like. A poly family is created with the members' own rules, style, and creativity. It can be as big or as small as desired, as long as the members are in consensus.

Polyamory is not just *Big Love* or niche reality TV anymore; it's a growing lifestyle. In fact, the very first International Academic Polyamory Conference occurred in February 2016 in Berkeley, California (not a surprise, given that Berkeley is one of the most politically and socially liberal cities in the country).

Adventurous V

More About Polyamory Love

* Poly people don't feel that something is *missing* from a current relationship when they bring in a secondary partner.
* Around thirty percent of the poly community considers one partner as their *primary* partner. The other seventy percent don't want to commit to a primary or secondary partner. Psychologist Bjarne Holmes, a specialist in romantic relationships, points out that many polys live in triads or quads, in the belief that one partner is not more important than another.
* Polyamorous relationships are considered to be committed and respectful. Within them is open communication—all factors in a healthy relationship.
* Many polyamorous relationships involve families. To date, there has not been enough research to point to any negative effects of polyamory families on children, but early research finds that it is not detrimental.

Whereas other pursuits of the adventurous V tend to be more sex driven, polyamory embraces the idea that one may love as many people as one feels compelled to love, while, at the same time, blending in with society.

The case for polyamory is one more argument for the idea that in today's world there is no such thing as a traditional family. Tradition? Tradition! [cue music] Tradition appears to be what you make it.

Sexual Fetish

There's that chuckle-inducing six-letter word: Fetish. It does seem like lately we're always reading about the fetish-ization of one thing or another—everything from food to fannies and Mid-Century Modern anything. For the record, Webster's Dictionary defines fetish as (1) a strong and unusual need or desire for something, (2) an object that is believed to have magical powers, and (3) **a need or desire for an object, body part, or activity for sexual excitement**. Bingo!

People with sexual fetishes need to touch, smell, look at, or engage in a fantasy with their desired object in order to function sexually alone or with a partner. Interestingly, and perhaps not surprisingly, boys and men are traditionally more prone to fetishes. As Beverly Hills psychologist Dr. Melissa Richman corroborates, "We know men have fetishes around women's panties and the vagina, but fetish with women is rarely talked about and a less likely occurrence. A man with a fetish for women's panties may want or feel control over a woman in thinking that he has control over a woman's vagina [via her panties]. This fantasy of dominance over a woman's vagina can become obsessive. There is the menstruation fetish, the hairy vagina fetish, pee fetish, as well as the fat vagina fetish."

So much for the breakdown of the panty fetish.

In a wider study, involving 150,000 male and female members of an Internet discussion group on fetishism, the erotic preferences broke down as follows:

Preferences for Non-genital Body Parts— 33% of the Group:

* Feet or Toes (a whopping 47%)
* Body Fluids, such as blood or urine (9%)
* Body Features, such as obesity, height, hair, muscle and body modifications such as tattoos and piercings (44%)

Preferences for Objects Associated with the Body— 30% of the Group:

* Footwear (34%)
* Clothing and Accessories worn on the legs and buttocks, such as stockings and skirts (33%)
* Costumes, and, less commonly, stethoscopes, wristwatches, and diapers (33%)

Fetish Preferences for Most of the Remaining 37% of the Group:

* Anasteemaphilia, the attraction to one because of a difference in height.
* Axillism, the act of using the armpit for sex.
* Coprophilia, a fetish for feces.
* Dacryphilia, the arousal from seeing tears in the eyes of a partner.
* Ecouteurism, sexual arousal from hearing others have sex.
* Emetophiliam, sexual arousal from vomit or vomiting.
* Endytophilia, the desire to keep one's clothes on during intercourse.

* Exhibitionism, an abnormal compulsion to expose the genitals with the intent of provoking sexual interest in the viewed.
* Formicophilia, a fetish for having small insects crawl on your genitals.
* Hybristophillia, sexual attraction and arousal from sex with criminals.
* Masophilia, sexual pleasure obtained from receiving punishment (physical or psychological).
* Nasophilia, sexual arousal derived from the sight, touch, licking or sucking of your partner's nose.
* Necrophilia, an erotic attraction to corpses.
* Sadism—the opposite of masophilia—sexual gratification gained through causing pain or degradation to others.
* Siderodromophilia, sexual arousal from riding on trains.

"Does Having a Fetish Make Me a Social Deviant?"

Short answer: No, *unless* the pattern of the erotic fetish is persistent and creates significant distress or impairment in social, occupational, or other vital areas of daily functioning. When that's the case, psychotherapy may be recommended. However, know that there are many fetishes that are harmless for a person or couple.

Dr. Melissa Richman maintains, "Overall, nothing is unhealthy unless it becomes disruptive to healthy functioning. However, people who engage in non-traditional sexual practices such as Swinging and sexual fetishism often report that they struggle to find therapists and medical professionals who don't view their behavior as deviant. Although consensual adult activities and porn involving fetishes do not constitute 'traditional' sexual behavior and sex play, they are not diagnosable as pathology. To diagnose as pathology, such behavior would have to meet the criteria of causing distress to self or harm to another."

Reminds me of the age-old saying, "You do what you want, as long as you don't hurt anybody."

A Toy Story

Molly, a petite 71-year old woman with piercing blue eyes and a thick mane of grey hair, had seen the death of the love of her life eight years earlier, a man she'd been with for forty years, until he was killed during a good Samaritan deed—hit while changing a tire for a stranger on the side of the road. Molly's been my patient for twenty years, and every visit she recalls a fond memory of a time she and her husband had together.

Recently, though, Molly was happily reunited with her high school sweetheart, now living in Florida. They were getting together every three weeks or so and she was having the time of her life, but, as she told me through giggles, her vagina had "been on lockdown for the last eight years! No action, except for speculum exams." She was thinking about having sex...soon, so her question to me was, "Now what?"

We talked about her choices—a dildo or dilator in between visits with her new love, just to, literally, open things up a bit. Molly's idea was to try a Persian cucumber in lieu of what seemed to her to be a much scarier prospect, plus cucumbers were readily available in the produce section of her local market. After a couple months of employing a very well-scrubbed, condom-encased 'cuke 4 times a week, at

thirty-minute intervals—usually while watching the news—
she was ready to move on to the real thing.

Sex Toys

For centuries, sex toys have been used to increase sexual
pleasure. Far from being taboo, sex toys are welcomed into
the bedrooms of more than 25% of adults surveyed from
around the world, and now constitute a $15 billion industry.
(Take that, Brookstone!) Tawdry stereotypes of sex toys are
passé, and in some cases, the business of sex toys has been
rebranded "sexual wellness."

Top sex toys for women:

* **Dildos.** Ever versatile, they can be made of rubber,
  plastic, glass, metal, or wood (and, infrequently, vegetable). Large, larger!, small, thick, thin, brown, purple,
  rainbow: the choice is yours! A dildo resembles a
  penis and may have many unique features to enhance
  sexual pleasure. Some are textured and/or curved in
  order to stimulate the G-spot, clitoris, or anus, and to
  provide other stimulatory benefits.
* **Vibrators.** I do find that my patients love their
  vibrators. Vibrators are available in a variety of styles,
  shapes, and intensities—powered by battery or power
  cords, or fully rechargeable. A vibrator exists for every
  sexual need.
* **Restraints.** Just what they sound like—handcuffs,
  blindfolds, masks, neckties, scarves, or anything else
  that might be used in bondage.

When passing sex toys between partners, such as vibrators shared between women, make sure that the dildo or

vibrator is properly cleaned with non-fragrant soap and warm water. Vaginal infections and STIs can easily be passed from partner to partner via those toys if you're not vigilant.

Want the good news on sex toys? Benefits for women include higher levels of sexual function and greater satisfaction with partners. The benefits are similar for men as well, including lower risks of heart disease, stroke, and diabetes—a good return on a relatively low cost investment, indeed.

Haven't we all had some sort of sexual fantasy? Maybe sex with Leonardo DiCaprio, or Diego the plumber, or a mom at your kid's school, or maybe it involved more than one person, a threesome—with or without your partner—or perhaps it simply involved you *watching*. You know what I mean. The point is that the Adventurous V has a place in this world and ought to be allowed to explore the boundaries of "acceptable." Because what exactly is "acceptable?" One of the only boundaries I can think of is an absence of harm, but then again, *my* definition of harm may not be the same as someone else's. And on and on we could go on the merry-go-round of human behavior, religious convention, and *politics*. I simply want to empower you to explore your sexual needs and desires without judgment and fear. Let your vagina drive for a change. No fear.

Now go out there...but be safe.

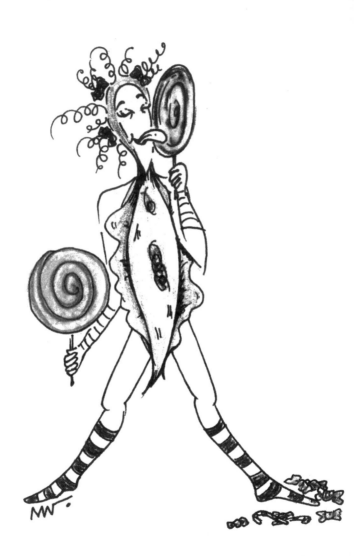

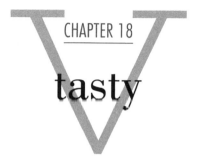

CHAPTER 18
tasty

66 Nothing, and I mean NOTHING is more terrifying for a lesbian on a date than the moment a girl is about to go down on her and she thinks to herself, "Oh God, please let it be safe down there." I realize straight women probably have this same fear...at least the ones I've slept with. I mean, I know we don't taste like mangos and strawberries—which is a good thing, otherwise I would be offering my lady parts to every attractive person I passed on the street: No, I'm serious! Just like mangos, you should check for yourself—but we always know when things aren't safe for visitors down there. Even with little to no time before I get down and dirty, I try and excuse myself just to clean up a little bit. I like to treat my vagina like a prizefighter who might be a little dazed and confused and not really sure what's about to happen after some hot foreplay. Splash a little water in her face, wake her up, and send her in!

She-ology

I've realized through my years of being a professional lesbian that the saying "we are what we eat" has truth to it. It's quite ironic, since most of the world knows what lesbians eat. We eat other lesbians. It's a vicious cycle. However, I found out that what we eat truly does affect the way we "taste" to other people. I remember going down on a girl who was taking at least twenty kinds of Chinese herbs to fight eczema. Let me tell you right now, it was the most distinct taste of Earth and Echinacea. If nothing else, I had a feeling my cold would be cured the minute she came. I had another experience where I was going down on a girl and she tasted incredibly sweet, but she was also incredibly sticky. "Did you accidentally spill pineapple juice on yourself?" I asked.

She laughed, "No, I read somewhere that pineapple is supposed to make you taste sweeter."

Before I went back to the task at hand, I calmly said, "Yes, I've heard that as well. But I think you're supposed to eat it." At least she was pretty.

Everyone is going to taste different. I was once told I tasted like candy. I almost felt bad for that poor woman. What kind of candy was she being fed as a child?! I've never had anyone come back up immediately after going downtown, so my vagina has either been palatable or I've dated some codependently polite women. I try and eat healthy and keep myself clean, but even with all my attention to detail there have been times when I thought to myself, "Oh, God, is that me?!" We all have that fear. It's normal. It's natural. What's *not* natural is sticking a douche up your vag because you saw a commercial about a mother and daughter playing volleyball on a beach and one of them had that "not so fresh feeling."

I think that Dr. Sherry will set you straight on all of this. Well, maybe wrong choice of words. It's not like she'll set you straight, but she'll *set you straight*, you know? She'll tell you how it is. 🍾🍾

—Dana Goldberg Comedian

Tasty V

I feel as if I've accomplished half my job as a gynecologist when a patient says to me, "Doc Sherry, you know what I love about you? I never feel weird telling you what's new with my vagina!" So started a recent conversation with my patient Lola. Several years ago, when Lola had her initial consultation, she began by asking, "Don't you find the vagina to be an enigma?" She had me laughing out loud in the first ten minutes. At twenty-nine, Lola is the epitome of a free-spirited SoCal gal. She's in touch, outspoken, and up for adventure. Lola left her dysfunctional family at seventeen and headed straight to Los Angeles to pursue her dream of being a comedienne. She put herself through a local college and landed her day job as a waitress in Venice Beach. On this recent visit she shared a story about her boyfriend, Nick: "Last time Nick and I had sex he told me, very diplomatically, that I tasted different lately. Okay, so after he left I was, like, dying to know what the hell he was talking about, and since I'm totally not gonna tie myself up into a freakin' pretzel to shove my face into my own bush, I did a finger test. And it did actually smell and taste pretty sour! I know you're not going to say I'm the first to tell you this kind of story, but I'm kind of freaking out. Obviously I'm clean down there, but what's the deal with the funky food taste?"

I will tell you what I told Lola: *You are what you eat* is an idiom for all things body-related. The connection is clear and apparent. Think about it: What happens when you eat asparagus? Within fifteen minutes your urine has that undeniably strange after-smell—actually this serves as the best example of how quickly food is broken down and excreted. After vitamins, your urine turns out bright green or yellow. Always (at least for me) the morning after eating beets you remind yourself, "It was the beets!" because for a moment you're sure that you're bleeding internally and have six months to live. If you're a smoker, nicotine is a detectable flavor in urine as well as sweat. Too much garlic the night before a big gym workout and you're reminded (in your perspiration) how garlic is the spice that keeps on giving. Pungent foods and spices seem to take a fast lane in our bodies through the blood stream, lungs, sweat, and vaginal secretions creating especially intense smells under arms, on the scalp, in the genital area... everywhere. Foods that may give off a notably offensive odor include: garlic, onions, mint, turmeric, curry, blue cheese and other fermented foods, cabbage, cauliflower, Brussels sprouts, broccoli, asparagus, vinegar, red meat and, perhaps, other foods such as eggs, liver, kidneys, seafood, fish oil, milk, peas, and soy!

The good news is that there are foods that can combat offensive odors and actually add a sweet smell or taste to the vagina. Take note of the groceries to have handy in your refrigerator:

* Fresh fruits (especially pineapple!)
* Fruit juices
* Vegetables (ones that are not aforementioned)
* Whole grains
* Greek yogurt
* Plenty of water

On any level—smell, taste, or general health-wise—nicotine is to be avoided, and alcohol and caffeine consumed in moderate amounts.

If your partner notices a different taste in your vaginal fluids, focus your first detective work on your diet. Has anything changed? Are you eating more beef, more fruits or vegetables, or are you focusing on one specific food group or single food (possibly in some new fad diet)? New medications, especially antibiotics, may factor in taste and smell changes. Rule of thumb: If a food gives you foul-smelling urine, farts, or breath, chances are it will affect the taste and smell of your vagina! After a thorough examination of possible dietary changes, I would suggest seeing your healthcare provider to eliminate the possibility of vaginal infection.

Odors: Other Culprits

Imagine: You're in the midst of a sexual encounter and your partner is passionately making their way down your body to get ready to give you oral sex—*to eat a peach, dine at the Y, get to third base, clean the kitchen, muff dive.* It's the moment before cunnilingus and you're suddenly outside your body, seized by the thought, "Oh, no, am I clean down there?!" You are in good company.

One statistic I came across stated that 72% of women are self-conscious about having an odor during oral sex. Apparently there is a website offering "Altoids for the vagina." How do I know this? A dear, *young* patient of mine ordered such product because she was so anxious about "smelling badly down south." She enthused that the minty pills helped ease her anxiety and gave her an extra "internal tingle." The only problem with the tingle was that it surfaced as the result of a raging yeast infection. When I used the speculum to see what was happening, I found two, small vaginal Altoids encased in clumps of white discharge. I made her promise to stick with the G-rated oral Altoids and rely on a little non-fragrant soap and water for some good old-fashioned odor protection.

She-ology

As explained more fully in Healthy V, a healthy vagina has a certain natural scent that is not unpleasant, and the arrival of an offensive, fishy, yeasty, or foul odor should signal a visit to your gynecologist to rule out a bacterial or yeast infection. With the help of thirty or so organisms working as a team, the healthy vagina maintains its **naturally acidic pH** and its natural, somewhat neutral smell. Anything that disrupts the natural pH balance, such as certain foods, spices, alcohol, caffeine, nicotine and medications, can affect the vagina's smell and taste, not to mention create a yeast or bacterial infection. Case in point: A diabetic who eats too much sugar is more prone to yeast infections. One of my longtime patients is an insulin-dependent diabetic, and I can tell if she's properly managing her glucose control by the frequency of her yeast infections!

Basic anatomy may be responsible for a new, unpleasant vaginal odor. Given that the urethra (where the urine comes out) sits directly above the vaginal opening, the smell of urine can definitely build up in the area. So with the clitoris sitting above the urethra, and the vagina as its neighbor below, it's a good (considerate) notion to clean your vagina before oral sex. That old urine can linger too close to the clitoris.

For married couples with routine sex dates (weekly, bimonthly or Saturday nights) it's a bit easier to prepare your body in a hygienic manner—*Hey, honey, I'll be ready at 10 p.m. sharp!* For those of you who maintain the spontaneity of different times and/or different partners, you can still take a moment to clean up. You and your partner will both be grateful (and relieved).

Tasty V

For more on how best to keep your vagina clean and healthy please see the chapter on the Healthy V! But for a quickie sum up, here are the simplest ways to keep a clean V:

* Practice daily hygiene, using non-fragrant soap or intimate wash and water on the vagina. And if you find yourself in a spontaneous sexual rendezvous, remember to make a quick vagina-readiness dash to a bathroom before getting naked.
* Wipe front to back, always
* Use probiotics to help keep the natural acidic pH balance of the vagina in check.
* Keep feminine hygiene wipes, just in case.

What NOT to do:

* Douche! (Douching is a sure way to disrupt the natural pH balance of the vagina and render it even *more* susceptible to infection and irritation.)
* Be sexually intimate if you haven't bathed or showered in the last 24 hours.
* Make a habit of chowing down on foods that result in offensive odors.

I am certainly not one to pussy shame anyone for their vagina smells—sweet, malodorous, or otherwise. I would simply advise you to keep check on keeping your lady parts clean, and to be aware of any changes in smell and taste. Don't be fooled by marketing ploys promising the freshest of vagina smells with the use of a spray, lube, cream, or juice. (Just say no to Freedom Spray, Massengill's Cleansing Tropical Breeze, Summer's Eve, Malibu Musk and Pussy Juice Vagina Flavoring.)

She-ology

Take my advice, and the advice of my trusted circle of fab women friends, non-fragrant soap or an intimate wash and water (and maybe a little less garlic and blue cheese) will keep your Tasty V appetizing...and happy.

ACKNOWLEDGEMENTS

Writing this book has been a dream of mine for many years.

I've always believed that anything, any dream in life is possible if you work hard and surround yourself with a *dream posse*, and I have been fortunate enough to have that posse in the form of inspiring, compassionate and loving friends, patients and family, so many of whom helped to make this book happen.

First I want to thank my patients. It is they who inspired the writing of this book, and it is their honesty, their humor and intelligent inquiry that make my job rewarding each and every day.

To those friends who helped add a special dimension to *She-ology*: Amy Acker, Christina Applegate, Meredith Baxter, Ashley Benson Naama Bloom, Wendy Burch, Jillian Dempsey, Gina Gershon, Dana Goldberg, Leisha Hailey, Lisa Gay Hamilton, Yolanda Hadid, Vicki Iovine, Louise Keoghan, Evelyn Lozada, Camryn Manheim, Debbie Matenopoulos, Katharine McPhee, Angela Nazarian, Kelly and Linda Novak, Kimberly Quaid, Jen Nicholson-Salke, Eden Sassoon, Jane Seymour, Brooke Shields, Shannon Tweed. It has been an honor to share in the intimate times of your lives—times that have been both wondrous and difficult—and I am so grateful for your contributions.

Special thanks to Reese Witherspoon for her inspiring, heartfelt introduction. Reese, your kindness and generosity of spirit are ever contagious.

Extra big thanks to those who pushed me to write this book and buoyed me along the path: Ann Hollister, Mary Connelly, Harriet Sternberg, Karen Rizzo, Danielle Tatum, Andrea Hartman, Lisa Heide-Ross, Gloria Acosta, your advice and support was invaluable.

Ana "Magumi" Wada, thank you for bringing my chapters to life with your beautiful and creative vagina caricatures.

To my sisters Brenda Daly, Johanna Daly, Veronica Gutierrez, Susannah Gutierrez, Polita Gutierrez, Debbie Battaglia, Jennifer Brown and Allison Enciso, I am grateful for you every day and especially so for your patience in reading my drafts!

Dr. Melissa Richman, Dr. Peter Loisides, Dr. Hal Danzer, Dr. Stephen Stein and Tamara Kline, thank you all. Your professional insight and contributions were invaluable in my research.

If there is such a thing as a goddess of serendipity, then it was she along with the enthusiastic Karen Kinney who brought me to my literary agent Nena Madonia. Nena has not only been a friend, she has championed this project from beginning to end and helped make it a labor of love.

To my sons, Michael, Stephen and Jonathan Becker, I am so proud of the young men you have become. You keep me hopeful for the future in your innate respect for women and your capacity for love.

To my wife and partner in love and life, Dr. Peggy Gutierrez, your unfailing support and unconditional love inspires and humbles me daily. I can only wonder: What do you do when your real life exceeds your dreams? Because that is exactly what has happened to me with you by my side.